D1757629

MILESTONES IN
LEUKEMIA RESEARCH AND THERAPY

Milestones in Leukemia Research and Therapy

EMIL J FREIREICH, M.D.
Ruth Harriet Ainsworth Professor of Developmental Therapeutics

NOREEN A. LEMAK, M.D.
Research Associate

Department of Hematology
The University of Texas
M. D. Anderson Cancer Center

The Johns Hopkins University Press   Baltimore and London

The Johns Hopkins University Press
701 West 40th Street, Baltimore, Maryland 21211
The Johns Hopkins Press Ltd., London

The paper used in this book meets the minimum requirements of American National Standards for Information Sciences—Permanence of Paper for Printed Library Materials, ANSI Z39.48-1984.

LIBRARY OF CONGRESS CATALOGING-IN-PUBLICATION DATA
Freireich, Emil J 1927–
    Milestones in leukemia research and therapy / Emil J Freireich and Noreen A. Lemak.
        p.   cm.—(The Johns Hopkins series in contemporary medicine and public health)
    Includes bibliographical references and index.
    ISBN 0-8018-4130-5 (alk. paper)
    1. Leukemia—History. 2. Leukemia—therapy. 3. Research—history. I. Lemak, Noreen A.   II. Title.   III. Series.
RC643.F725   1991
616.99'419—dc20
DNLM/DLC
for Library of Congress   90-5362

We shall not cease from exploration.
And the end of all our exploring
Will be to arrive where we started
And know the place for the first time.

T. S. ELIOT (1888–1965), "Little Gidding" in *Four Quartets*

Contents

Preface

Another damned, thick, square book!
Always scribble, scribble, scribble!
Eh! Mr. Gibbon?

WILLIAM HENRY, DUKE OF GLOUCESTER (1743–1805),
upon receiving from Edward Gibbon volume 2 of
The Decline and Fall of the Roman Empire (1781)

We started writing a brief review of leukemia and ended up with a book! The project was undertaken because we could find no historic discussion of leukemia that covered the events from 1940 to the present, even though the knowledge of leukemia has advanced more during the last 50 years than during all prior centuries.

Research in hematologic malignancies has been the vanguard of cancer investigation, and many consider that the control of leukemia will be the key to unlocking the mystery of the control of other malignant disease in humans. Leukemia research has been likened to the bow of the ship—always plunging ahead first to break uncharted waters, while the rest of the craft follows behind. This is understandable because blood is readily available for monitoring responses in experimental investigations. One cannot easily take intermittent samples of a kidney tumor, but repeated examination of blood presents no problem. Also, acute leukemia is a systemic stage IV disease virtually from its onset;

it was therefore an appropriate choice for pioneering studies of systemic chemotherapeutic agents.

Many life-saving advances in oncology were researched and developed first in mice bearing transplantable leukemias and then in human patients with leukemia. The list of the resulting benefits includes most of the chemotherapeutic agents and combinations of agents; blood transfusions; platelet and leukocyte transfusions; many antibacterial and antifungal agents, especially those for neutropenic patients; protected environmental units; gut-sterilizing regimens; many of the biologic response modifiers; bone marrow transplantation; and the major part of the work to date in cytogenetics. Avery Sandberg noted that, "though tumors make up the bulk of human neoplasia, cytogenetically they represent a small percentage of available chromosome data in human neoplasia, with the leukemias dominating overwhelmingly."[1]

In writing this book, we chose to go back to the original articles whenever possible and allow the authors' own words to tell the story. Therefore, we have included many quotations. Also, to avoid any misunderstanding in descriptions of clinical protocols and results of trials, we tried to use the precise terms of the investigators. Admittedly, some subjects are treated in a sketchy manner, but extensive references are provided to guide those who want more information.

Some readers may regard the many pages devoted to chemotherapeutic agents as excessive. From our viewpoint, however, the major part of the history of leukemia since 1940 is embodied in the search for and the development of antileukemic therapy. We hope that physicians who use these drugs will be interested to read details about the discovery and evolution of the substances.

Over the years, pivotal events stood out as momentous milestones that served to stimulate an entire discipline, and we have attempted to highlight these episodes. Such happenings were the trial of aminopterin in childhood leukemia by Farber and colleagues (1948), the discovery of the structure of DNA by Watson and Crick (1953), the first combination chemotherapy trials (late 1950s and early 1960s), the citing of the corrected number of human chromosomes by Tjio and Levan (1956), the discovery of the Ph[1] chromosome by Nowell and Hungerford (1960), and the synthesis of the first recombinant DNA molecules at Stanford

University (1972). Many equally important advances, however, took place over many years, for example, the work of physicians at the National Cancer Institute (in the 1950s and 1960s) that culminated in procedures such as platelet and leukocyte transfusions to aid in controlling hemorrhage and infection in patients undergoing antileukemic therapy, Bodey's successes in preventing and managing infections, and the accomplishments of the Seattle group in bone marrow transplantation. A review of the background issues that set the stage for the achievements of these investigators will furnish, we hope, an appropriate and accurate perspective.

As the chapters kept expanding, we could sympathize with Geoffrey Fisher, Archbishop of Canterbury, who, after receiving suggestions that more saints should be canonized in the Church of England, complained, "Once you start, there is no end to who is to go in and who is to be left out."[2] We heartily applaud and apologize sincerely to all those dedicated researchers whose life work went unmentioned.

Many of our readers may be senior physicians (like ourselves) whose only background in genetics was a brief acquaintance with the work of Gregor Mendel. Therefore, in the passages on cytogenetics and molecular genetics we tried to define terms and provide a simplified description of some of the more sophisticated experimental research. Persons who work in these areas will undoubtedly find parts of the text too elementary.

An author's effort to write a work of history, said Erwin Chargaff, "must be very difficult as long as some of the witnesses, with all their quirks, senilities and dubious recollections are still alive. Later it will be easier . . . no one being left to protest against truth or falsehood."[3]

We are grateful to our colleagues at the University of Texas M. D. Anderson Cancer Center for their assistance, especially Gerald P. Bodey, M.D., for his invaluable help with chapter 6 and Tao-Chiuh Hsu, Ph.D., for his suggestions to improve chapter 8. We also thank Barbara H. Reschke of the Department of Scientific Publications for her advice.

This endeavor was supported in part by National Institutes of Health Grant No. CA39809 and by the Ruth Harriet Ainsworth Chair for Research.

ONE

Before the Twentieth Century

Physicians of the utmost fame
Were called at once; but when they came
They answered, as they took their fees,
"There is no cure for this disease."

HILAIRE BELLOC (1870–1953), "Physicians of Utmost Fame"

Velpeau

The first documented description of a case of leukemia was probably that of a French surgeon, Alfred Velpeau, in 1827.[1,2] Dameshek and Gunz described the case.

> His patient, a 63-year-old florist and seller of lemonade, who had abandoned himself to the abuse of spirituous liquor and of women without, however, becoming syphilitic, fell ill in 1825 with a swelling of the abdomen, fever, and weakness. He died soon after admission to the hospital and was at autopsy found to have an enormous liver and spleen, the latter weighing ten pounds. The blood was thick, like gruel . . . resembling in consistency and color the yeast of red wine. . . . One might have asked if it were not rather laudable pus, mixed with blackish coloring matter, than blood.[2]

Velpeau asked, "Does the condition of the spleen and liver cause the decomposition of the blood, or, could it be that the abnormal fluid produces the enlargement of these organs?"[3]

Further enlightenment did not come until the advent of microscopy in medical training. Antonj van Leeuwenhoek was examining his own blood with a primitive microscope in 1673, but almost two centuries passed before the instrument's value to medicine was recognized. During that lag period, medicine was rigidly controlled, and innovations from outside the organized network were restricted. Persons opposing the microscope spoke of "optical illusion," and this expression delayed for many years the introduction of microscopy to the study of medicine.[4]

Donné

Alfred Donné was a true pioneer when, in 1837, he organized a course in clinical microscopy despite the active opposition of his colleagues and of the Parisian medical faculty. Many students attended Donné's lectures and demonstrations, and he soon acquired a wide reputation. In 1839, he was asked to examine a postmortem blood sample from a woman who had suffered with a large abdominal tumor and diarrhea. Dr. Donné's analysis follows.

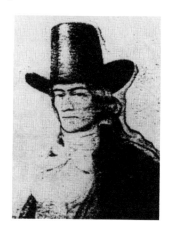

Alfred Francois Donné

The blood you sent me, my dear colleague, shows a remarkable change and, most conspicuous, despite the fact that it had been collected under unfavorable conditions, id est, from a dead body. More than half of the cells were "mucous globules." This fact needs perhaps some explanation. You know that normal blood contains three types of cells: 1. Red cells—the essential cellular constituent of the blood. 2. White cells or mucous cells (which I consider as being secreted from the vascular wall). 3. The small globules.

It is the second variety which dominates so much, that one wonders, knowing nothing about the clinical course, whether this blood does not contain pus. As you know, the pus cell cannot yet be differentiated, with definite accuracy, from mucous cells.[4]

In 1844, Donné reported on a case in which the blood had been collected in vivo.

There are conditions in which the white cells seem to be in excess in the blood. I found this fact so many times, it is so evident in certain patients, that I cannot conceive the slightest doubt in this regard. One can find in some patients such a great number of these cells, that even the least experienced observer is greatly impressed. I had an opportunity of seeing these in a patient on the service of Dr. Rayer at the Hôpital de la Charité. This man, who was in the prime of life, was affected with arteritis, especially in the vessels of his legs. Both legs were the site of ecchymoses, gangrenous blisters. The blood of this patient showed such a number of white cells that I thought that his blood really was mixed with pus, but at the end I was unable to observe a clear-cut difference between these cells and the white cells. At autopsy there was no trace of pus in the vessels or in the interior of the clots.[4]

Donné reported this case in his treatise on microscopy,[5] published in 1844, and is credited with the first known observation of leukemia. For the first time in medical history, leukemia was associated with hematologic abnormality.[6]

Bennett versus Virchow

Among Donné's pupils was a young Scottish physician, John Hughes Bennett.[7] In 1845, Bennett and the German pathologist Rudolph Virchow each published a case history of a patient whose autopsy findings included marked enlargement of the spleen. Bennett's patient had experienced symptoms for 21 months and had widespread lymphatic tumors as well as hypertrophy of the liver and spleen.[8] Virchow's patient was admitted to the hospital with loss of weight, severe coughing, swelling of the lower extremities, and frequent bloody stools. She developed severe epistaxis and died 5 months later.[4,9] Bennett observed that "the following case seems to me particularly valuable, as it will serve to demonstrate the existence of true pus, formed universally within the vascular system."[10] Virchow did not attempt to explain the abnormal findings. He noted that previous accounts of white blood related mostly to loss of blood by hemorrhage, fasting, etc., and that these reports

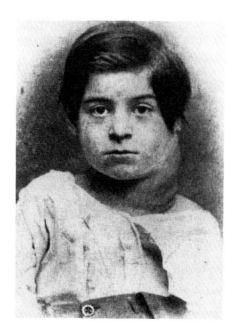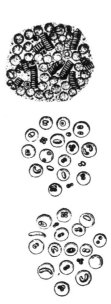

(Left) *First photograph of a patient with leukemia, 1862.* (Right) *Microscopic appearance of blood in a case of leukemia reported by Bennett JH: Case of hypertrophy of the spleen and liver, in which death took place from suppuration of the blood.* Edinburgh Med Surg J *64:413–423, 1845; and* Leucocythemia, or White Cell Blood, *Edinburgh, Sutherland and Knox, 1852.*

were "quite useless because microscopic examination was lacking."[4]

These two publications appeared within 1 month of each other, and the young authors (Bennett, age 33; Virchow, age 24) entered into a prolonged dispute over who was first with the correct interpretation. The quarrel escalated as many prominent physicians in several countries took sides; medical meetings and literature over the next 50 years were tainted by this controversy.

In 1846, Virchow took issue with Bennett's belief that the blood's light color indicated a general pyemia,[10] and in an 1847 publication Virchow described his second case and concluded that the blood disease he named "leukämie" was a pathologic entity

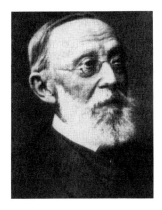

Rudolf Virchow

by itself and not a symptomatic suppuration of the blood.[11] He defined leukemia as "an increase in the number of colorless blood corpuscles to the extent that the red color of blood turns into reddish, yellowish, or greenish white."[10] He was now convinced that changes in the spleen and in the lymphatic glands caused changes in the blood's composition: "For the time being, one has to presume that leukemia is a primary autonomous disease of the spleen and the lymphatic glands and the direct cause for the increase in the number of colorless particles in the blood."[10,11]

Virchow reported his third case of leukemia in 1849[12] and, on the basis of these three examples, reached a final judgment that there were two types of leukemia, namely, a splenic and a lymphatic form.[10,13] The former "brings elements into the blood that are analogous to the components of the spleen's pulpa," whereas the latter "provides elements analogous to the parenchymatous granules of the lymphatic glands."[10,14] This was the earliest attempt to classify leukemias, but Virchow still believed that red cells constituted the normal end stage in the development of all blood cells and that the white corpuscles were immature, not yet having acquired the red color.[10]

Vogel

In 1854, Dr. Julius Vogel, a Professor of Medicine at the University of Giessen (Germany), published the first paper describing in detail the clinical picture ("The Symptomatology of Leukemia").[3] He wrote the chapter "Storungen der Blutmischung" ("Disturbances of the Contents of the Blood") in the first volume of Virchow's *Handbuch*. Vogel's paper is based on observation of 25 patients (16 male and 9 female). The author, who proudly claimed to have been the first in Germany to make the diagnosis of leukemia in vivo, described the illness as a chronic disease with a slow, insidious onset and a progressive, fatal course. He listed the following signs and symptoms: fatigue, general malaise, diarrhea, sometimes coughing and dyspnea, fever, intensive pallor, enlargement of spleen and liver; in some cases, the outstanding finding is enlargement of the lymphatics. Like Velpeau, he speculated: "Is the blood alteration a consequence of engorgement of spleen and lymph nodes or is it the other way? Is the excessive amount of white cells the primary lesion which causes enlargement of the spleen and lymphatics?"[3]

Friedreich

Nikolaus Friedreich, at age 31, had succeeded his mentor, Virchow, in the chair of pathologic anatomy at Würzburg.[15] In 1857, Friedreich described a 46-year-old woman with weakness, hemorrhages, oral ulceration, and hepatosplenomegaly developing rather rapidly over a period of about 5 weeks.[16] She died 5 days after admission to the hospital. The final pathologic diagnosis of the case was an acute form of leukemia. Friedreich based this on two findings: the spleen was soft and flaccid, whereas it had been solid in all cases previously described, and the number of white corpuscles in the circulating blood had not yet progressed to the degree seen in earlier cases. This was the first report of acute leukemia.[10]

Dameshek and Gunz summarized this first phase of research on leukemia by stating that, within 12 years of its recognition, the two chief varieties of chronic leukemia, as well as the acute form, had been described and the main clinical and pathologic features had been recorded.[2] Owing to the crude hematologic methods then available, it was possible to make only the most superficial examination of leukocytes, and they could not be characterized morphologically or traced back to the sites of their formation. It had been realized, however, that the changes in the blood were caused not by a mixture of pus but probably by a rapid production of those white corpuscles that are a normal constituent of blood. The primary abnormalities in the disease were now sought in the "lymphatic organs" rather than in the blood itself.[2]

Even at this time, there were still many irreconcilable opponents who denied the very existence of leukemia.[2] At a medical meeting in Paris in 1855, Cahen[17] stated that "leukemia has no special causes, special symptoms, particular anatomic lesions or specific treatment, and I thus conclude that it does not exist as a distinct malady."[2] Another researcher (Barthez)[18] added, "There are enough diseases without inventing any new ones."[2]

Woodward

The final 40 years of the nineteenth century brought several momentous additions to the accumulated knowledge of leukemia. The foremost American histopathologist of this period was Joseph Janvier Woodward, who had performed the autopsy on President Lincoln and who later attended President Garfield during the interval between his wounding and his death. Woodward was very active in the Civil War and wrote two volumes of *The Medical and Surgical History of the War of the Rebellion* (1861–65), which he prepared in accordance with acts of Congress. His studies in pathology marked the beginning in the United States of objective research into the nature of neoplastic disease, a field then dominated by European medicine led by Virchow.[19] In addition, Woodward was the first person to use aniline dyes in histology (1865),[20] and these were to aid greatly in the differentiation of white blood cells.[10]

Neumann

In 1870, Ernst Neumann reported changes in the bone marrow in a 30-year-old man who had died from splenic leukemia.[21] "The marrow in the central cavity of the humerus and in the retiform spaces of the so-called spongy bones (ribs, sternum, one thoracic vertebra) was of the same greenish-yellow color that I already mentioned to have found also in the diploe of the cranium, and its consistency was that of a very viscous pus."[10] Neumann surmised that there might be a "myelogenous" leukemia in addition to the splenic and lymphatic forms.[2] His meticulous studies on the function of bone marrow continued over many years, and in 1878 he wrote that all leukemias had their origin in the bone marrow.[10,22] According to Rauscher and Shimkin,[23] M. A. Novinsky, a Russian veterinarian, transplanted two cancers into dogs in 1877, but this attracted little attention.

Gowers

In a comprehensive monograph (1880),[24] Sir William Gowers pointed out that the anemia that is one of the important findings in leukemia might be due to an accelerated destruction of red cells, not just their slowed formation.[10] He also believed that the increase in the number of white cells in the blood was only a symptom accompanying the primary changes in the blood-forming organs and that it need not be present before the diagnosis of leukemia could be established.[2] He thus anticipated the later recognition of the aleukemic forms of leukemia.

Ehrlich

Paul Ehrlich (1891)[25] used various dyes (first introduced by Woodward) to develop intricate staining methods in an effort to classify the different white blood cells as appropriate to either the spleen or the bone marrow. Unexpectedly, he found that he could not differentiate. Seufert and Seufert stated that "one would have to conclude from this absolutely identical behavior of all cells containing polymorphous nuclei that, contrary to previously held beliefs, the bone marrow and spleen produce the same colorless blood elements. Thus, when classified according to the origin of white blood cells, only two systems existed, namely, the lymphatic and the myeloic (myelogenous) systems."[10]

Thus, the term *splenic leukemia* was dropped from the nomenclature,[10] and the former method of categorization based on gross anatomic lesions of lymph nodes and spleen was displaced.[26] Ehrlich is regarded as the founder of the discipline of hematology because, with his differential staining techniques, he described eosinophils, basophils, and neutrophils and demonstrated that leukemia could be diagnosed by a blood smear.[27] He was able to trace the origin of the granular cells back to a precursor cell, the *myelocyte*.[28] Ehrlich was awarded the Nobel Prize in chemistry in 1908.

Naegeli

Naegeli (1900)[29] described cells in the marrow that resembled "large lymphocytes" and created the name *myeloblast*.[28] His studies led to the concept that the two main forms of leukemia were generalized in nature.[26] Carl O. Jensen, a Danish veterinarian, reported tumor transplantation in mice (1903).[23] "His work attracted immediate attention because mice in which transplants grew and then regressed were found to be immune to further transplants."[23]

Auer

In 1906, John Auer described rods in the cytoplasm of "large lymphocytes" in a blood smear taken from a 21-year-old man with acute leukemia. The patient had been admitted to Dr. Osler's wards at Johns Hopkins on April 25, 1903, and died May 16 of that year.[30] A short paper by Reschad and Schilling-Torgau in 1913 reported a new form of acute leukemia in which the monocyte was considered to be the malignant cell.[31]

The list now included chronic lymphocytic, chronic granulocytic (myelogenous), acute lymphocytic, acute granulocytic (myeloblastic), and acute monocytic leukemias.[2] Thus, the stage was finally set, at the beginning of the twentieth century, for research into the etiology of leukemia and for the development of useful therapies.

In the following chapters, the terms "granulocytic leukemia" and "myelogenous leukemia" will be used interchangeably, as we will conform to the usage of different authors.

TWO

Etiology

We dance round in a ring and suppose,
But the Secret sits in the middle and knows.

ROBERT FROST (1874–1963), "The Secret Sits"

Furth and Kahn

Researchers have been "supposing" about the cause of leukemia for many decades, and evidence seems to indicate a complex etiology. A vast array of fundamental knowledge has been well documented. A good choice to begin the list of investigations into etiology is a truly landmark article describing research in an appropriate strain of mice by Furth and Kahn (1937), showing that "a single malignant white blood cell is capable of producing the systemic disease—leukemia—which has hitherto been regarded by many workers as having a multicentric origin."[1] Today, clonal selection is generally accepted as the "process by which cancer develops and evolves."[2]

VIRUSES

Ellermann and Bang

In 1903, Borrel[3] suggested that cancer is caused by a virus,[4] but the first substantial breakthrough concerning the etiology of leukemia came in May 1908, when Ellermann and Bang[5] reported that chicken leukemia could be transmitted by filtrates and was, presumably, caused by a virus.[6] Many skeptics were uneasy with this conclusion and, although finally forced to accept the facts, believed that virus-caused leukemia occurred only in chickens.[6]

Gross

Forty-three years passed before Gross (1951)[7] demonstrated in mice that leukemia could be transmitted by filtered extracts, proving that leukemia is caused by a virus in mammals, too. As he summarized:

> Mouse leukemia is due to a submicroscopic, leukemogenic virus, . . . which is transmitted from one generation to another directly through the embryos. The virus remains in most instances latent, causing leukemia only when activated, usually in animals which reach or pass five to six months of age. The nature of the trigger factors causing activation of the virus is obscure. Usually, the activating factors are internal, presumably of metabolic or hormonal origin. Some trigger factors may also be external, such as carcinogenic chemicals or radiation energy.[6]

The evidence that viruses cause chicken and mouse leukemia naturally aroused workers worldwide to search for a similar cause of human leukemia. Over the years, many electron microscopists have seen virus-like particles, but, of course, these findings could not be taken as proof that the particles were the cause of cancer.[8] Therefore, the discovery of a retrovirus occurring in humans was a landmark, and circumstances contributing to that successful culmination are interesting.

HTLV-I

In 1960, Nowell[9] discovered that lymphocytes could be activated or stimulated to enter a proliferative cycle by adding lectins, such as phytohemagglutinins, to the culture medium.[10] Subsequently, it was learned that the cells being activated were the T lymphocytes, and, unfortunately, it was not possible to maintain T cell proliferation.[10] Then Morgan et al. (1976)[11] reported selective growth of T lymphocytes when unfractionated normal human bone marrow cells were cultured with conditioned medium obtained from phytohemagglutinin-stimulated normal human lymphocytes. Cultures up to 90 percent T cells had been maintained for more than 9 months. They found that the T cell secreted a protein that sustained proliferation; the protein was termed T cell growth factor (TCGF).[10] This was later called interleukin 2.

After the discovery of reverse transcriptase in 1970, methodic investigations were started in search of evidence for low-level expression of a human retrovirus.[10] (The genetic material in a retrovirus is RNA [ribonucleic acid]; the reverse transcriptase enzyme is associated with the translation of RNA into DNA [desoxyribonucleic acid] so that replication can take place. The virus is called "retro" because the transfer of genetic information is "backward.") The first detection of human T cell leukemia virus (HTLV) was achieved (Poiesz et al., 1980[12,13]) by growing neoplastic T cells (from certain patients) with TCGF in suspension cultures and examining the media for particle-associated reverse transcriptase. This was validated by electron microscopic studies.[10] The first isolates were prepared in the United States from adult black patients with aggressive forms of T cell malignancy. Many additional isolates have come from patients in the Caribbean, Japan, Africa, South America, and Israel. These all belong to the same subgroup of virus HTLV-I.[10]

HTLV-II

Kalyanaraman and colleagues (1982)[14] reported a new subtype of human T cell leukemia virus (HTLV-II) associated with a T cell variant of hairy cell leukemia.

HTLV-III

During 1983 and 1984, three laboratories independently isolated the retrovirus believed responsible for acquired immunodeficiency syndrome (AIDS).[15-18] The virus was given three different names, one by each group of investigators. It was labeled *human T-lymphotropic virus (HTLV-III), lymphadenopathy-associated virus (LAV),* and *AIDS-related virus (ARV).*[19] Researchers suspected that these were all the same virus, but the genetic codes had to be determined and compared.[19]

By 1985, the genetic code had been clarified by Ratner et al.[20] and, subsequently, the virus has been named human immunodeficiency virus (HIV). According to Wong: "Shortly thereafter, it was discovered that viruses recovered from an individual over time have minor genetic variations, and more than one virus (although very similar in genetic sequence) had been isolated as the causative agent for AIDS.[21] These discoveries have increased the difficulties in developing a vaccine and finding a cure for the disease."[19] It has recently been reported that "the minor degree of HIV sequence heterogeneity which occurs within a given infected individual may be sufficient to allow the virus to evade an ongoing T cell response. . . . Even one conservative substitution can drastically reduce recognition."[22]

Human T cell leukemia virus is the only retrovirus known to occur in humans. Evidence suggests that HTLV-III is a virus that can cause target cells to both proliferate (leukemia) and be depleted (immunosuppression).[23] Clinically, infection with this retrovirus presents as an opportunistic infection or a neoplasm, such as Kaposi's sarcoma or B cell lymphoma.[19]

RADIATION

The first report that overexposure to x-rays could result in leukemia was by von Jagić et al. (1911)[24]; they described the occurrence of leukemia in four persons who had had prolonged exposure to radiation.[25] Their article was followed by many anecdotal accounts of leukemia among persons receiving small doses of radiation over prolonged periods. March listed 13 such papers in the bibliography accompanying his 1944 publication, "Leukemia in Radiologists."[25] Since there had been no known statistical study of the problem, March reviewed all physician death notices from radiology journals and the *Journal of the American Medical Association* between 1929 and 1943. He determined that leukemia was the cause of death in 8 of 175 radiologists who succumbed during that period, an incidence of 4.57 percent. Among nonradiologic physicians, the incidence of death from leukemia was 0.44 percent. Thus, leukemia occurred in radiologists more than 10 times as often as in other physicians.[25]

Hiroshima and Nagasaki

The largest single collection of data on radiation leukemia is that gathered from the survivors of the atomic bomb.[26-30] After single large explosions at Hiroshima (August 6, 1945) and Nagasaki (August 9, 1945), many persons developed severe aplasia of the bone marrow. In those who recovered, there was a definite increase in the incidence of leukemia, which seemed to commence about 18 months after the bombing. The largest number of cases appeared in 1951–52.[26] Because these persons had a one-time flash exposure to the rays, the incubation period could be ascertained quite specifically.

In the first report of a case of leukemia in an A-bomb survivor, Misao et al. (1953)[27] described a 19-year-old man who had been exposed at a distance of 1,000 meters from the hypocenter in Nagasaki. Although he had recovered after a moderate acute phase, 3 months later he again showed signs of high fever, sore throat, and subcutaneous hemorrhage and was diagnosed as suffering from acute monocytic leukemia.[28] Among the A-bomb survivors of Hiroshima, the first reported case of acute leukemia was that of a 27-year-old man who was diagnosed 14 months after exposure.[28,29]

The incidence of leukemia was particularly high in people exposed to more than 1 Gy (100 rad). Although it declined in this population during the 1960s, the incidence between the years 1965 and 1971 was still elevated, at 25.35 per 100,000 population. The death rate from leukemia during the same period in Japan was approximately 3.3 per 100,000 population; therefore, the incidence of leukemia among those exposed to large doses of radiation was more than seven times higher.[28]

The risk of leukemia diminished with elapsed time, but there are no indications that the risk has returned to control levels in those who received a significant dose of radiation, even 30 years after the bombings.[30] Fortunately, there seems to be no discernible genetic damage in the children of the Japanese survivors.[31]

As Gunz (1977) wrote in 1977:

When the leukaemogens are considered as a body, it becomes clear that those now known or suspected to be active in man can account for only a part, and probably a small part, of the cases which occur sporadically in any one population . . . even the most powerful agent produces disease in only a small proportion of those exposed to it. Thus the leukaemia incidence among those A-bomb victims closest to the hypocentre of the explosion was little more than one per cent, even though it exceeded that among the unexposed by nearly 60 times in Hiroshima and 30 times in Nagasaki. Clearly those who developed leukaemia must have had a heightened personal predisposition which the majority of the radiation-exposed population lacked.[32]

Therapeutic Radiation

Court-Brown and Doll (1965) reviewed 14,554 patients with ankylosing spondylitis whose therapy included radiation given during the period 1935 to 1954. Follow-up averaged 13 years, with a maximum of 25 years. Fifty-two deaths from leukemia were recorded; 5.48 was the expected number of deaths from leukemia. Thus, there were 9.5 times as many deaths in the irradiated patients as expected. Deaths from leukemia increased over the first 5 years of follow-up and then declined.[33]

CHEMICALS

Soot

Sir Percival Pott, the eminent eighteenth-century surgeon of London's St. Bartholomew's Hospital, is the acknowledged first source of our information about chemical carcinogens.[34] In 1775, he reported an occupational cancer in his publication, *Chirurgical Observations Relative to the Cataract, the Polypus of the Nose, the Cancer of the Scrotum, the different kinds of ruptures, and the mortification of the toes and feet.*[35,36] His description of scrotal cancer in chimneysweeps leaves no doubt that the malady was recognized as being the result of chronic exposure to an environmental agent, soot, in youngsters whose fate was "singularly hard"[34] even for those days. The affliction was called "soot-wart" by those in the trade.[34] Soot-wart is a highly malignant squamous cell carcinoma.[37]

Benzene

This seems to be the chemical most frequently accused of causing leukemia. Since Selling's experiments with benzene in 1910,[38] we have known that it can cause damage to bone marrow.

Pioneer researchers suggested that benzene and the related chemicals toluene and xylene may cause leukemia in humans.[39] The first published report of leukemia in a benzol worker was that of Delore and Borgomano in 1928.[40] Lignac (1932)[41] induced leukocytic proliferation in mice by prolonged administration of benzene.[39]

Since that time, much evidence has accumulated to support the relation of chronic benzene exposure to leukemia. Dameshek's experience showed that

> the leukemia found is usually subacute. Cases have been observed in automobile mechanics exposed for years to various types of gases and oils, in persons working with oils and greases and using benzene and xylene for "cleaning up" and in those working with paint removers containing aromatic solvents and the like. Whether or not the leukemia is actually induced by the chemical is always in question in a given case, even when the exposure is clear-cut and prolonged.[39]

There is also a high incidence of leukemia after the application of certain hydrocarbons to the skin of mice. Morton and Mider (1938)[42] are given credit for the earliest report of this finding. They used a mouse strain that had been maintained for more than 25 generations in which leukemia occurred rarely and never before the animals were 18 months old. Forty-eight mice were used, and when they were 4 to 6 weeks old the researchers began painting the skin of each mouse. The material used was 0.5 percent methylcholanthrene (a petroleum hydrocarbon) in commercial benzene. It was applied with a brush, and the site was changed with each application so that the same area was not painted twice during a month. When the animals had received their 10th painting (69th day), a subcutaneous inguinal mass was found in a female. Three days later, bilateral inguinal and axillary lymphadenopathy was present. She died on the 75th day of the experiment. At autopsy, the axillary, inguinal, abdominal, and tracheobronchial nodes were greatly enlarged; the liver was pale with marked leukemic infiltration, and the spleen was large and gray and had lost normal structure. Nine more mice subsequently developed the same picture of widespread lymphomatosis. Blood studies on two mice revealed leukocytes numbering 90,000 and 139,000, respectively.[42]

Latta and Davies (1941) found that repeated daily subcutaneous injections of a benzene-olive oil mixture in rats produced a primary stimulation of the neutrophilic granulopoietic system followed by rapid destruction of circulating leukocytes. With heavy doses, the marrow became completely aplastic after 60 days, practically all lymphatic tissue had disappeared from spleen and lymph nodes, blood lymphocytes were reduced by 97 to 98 percent, and none of them were normal.[43]

In 1967, Forni and Moreo reported a detailed cytogenetic study of a patient who developed leukemia after 22 years of continuous exposure to benzene.[44] Sequential analyses were performed over a period of 15 months during which the disease progressed from aplastic anemia, with no immature cells in the peripheral blood, to a leukemic condition characterized by peripheral blood myeloblasts. Before immature cells appeared in the blood, hyperdiploid cells, each with 47 chromosomes, were detected in the bone marrow. When a frankly leukemic picture emerged, hyperdiploid cells from blood or bone marrow consistently contained an extra group C chromosome.[45] As Dean noted, the fact "that prolonged exposure to high concentrations of benzene results in myelotoxicity is beyond doubt, but the great differences in individual susceptibility to this hazard remain unexplained. It appears likely that other environmental factors in addition to benzene exposure are involved in the development of leukemia."[45]

Although many other chemicals produce chromosomal changes of a nonspecific nature, only a few chemicals have been branded as carcinogenic. Data seem to indicate that these chemicals do not require any alteration of the chromosomal set from diploidy to induce the neoplastic state. Neoplasia can occur just as readily in the presence of a diploid set of chromosomes.[46]

GENETICS

Videbaek

The first large study of familial leukemia was that of Videbaek (1947).[47] He collected data from a group of 209 patients with leukemia and their families and also from a cohort of 200 control families. Videbaek found that, if leukemia occurred in siblings, it developed when they were about the same age, making "fortuitous coincidence" unlikely.[39] The occurrence of several cases of leukemia in the same family was much too frequent to be explained by coincidence. More than 1 case of leukemia occurred in 17 of the 209 affected families, but there was only 1 case among all families of the control group;[48] the incidence was 8 versus 0.5 percent.

Videbaek also found that the incidence of cancers was much higher in relatives of leukemic patients than in control families, which supported speculation that a gene common to all types of neoplastic disease could be inherited. He finally concluded that the inheritance of leukemia was one of "predisposition" and that some other environmental agent was essential for the disease to develop.[39]

Inherited Syndromes

In humans, further evidence indicative of an inherited factor in leukemia and lymphoma comes from studies of inherited syndromes (ataxia-telangiectasia, Bloom's syndrome, Fanconi anemia) that include a susceptibility to leukemia and lymphoma. "While these account for only a small proportion of all cases of leukaemia, they demonstrate beyond all doubt that, in man, the process of leukaemogenesis is subject to genetic variability."[49] These conditions "may reflect an inherited gene defect present in all cells of the body."[50] Apparently, an abnormality of DNA repair processes exists, greatly increasing the likelihood of an abnormal clone and, eventually, a malignancy.[50]

In 1930, Brewster and Cannon[51] reported that leukemia had been diagnosed in an infant with Down's syndrome.[4] Stewart et al. (1958) wrote that among 677 children with acute leukemia, the number having Down's syndrome was 20 times that expected.[52]

Philadelphia Chromosome

Before the 1970s, articles on the genetic aspect of leukemia were sparse, but in recent years cytogenetics has flourished and the list of publications related to chromosomes and leukemia fills many columns in *Index Medicus*.

Although Boveri (1902)[53] suggested that malignant tumors could be due to an abnormal chromosome composition,[54] the true starting point can be identified as 1960, when Nowell and Hungerford

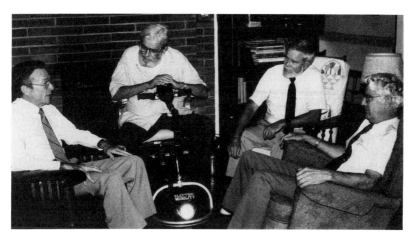

Left to right: *Warren Nichols, David Hungerford, Paul Moorhead, Peter Nowell. All were active in chromosome and lymphocyte culture work in Philadelphia in the early 1960s.*

described an abnormally small chromosome in the leukemic cells of two patients with chronic granulocytic leukemia (CGL).[55] Peter Nowell recalled:

> I joined the University of Pennsylvania faculty in 1956 and began culturing human leukemic cells using Edwin Osgood's method.[56] (This used phytohemagglutinin to get rid of the erythrocytes. . . .) Being trained in pathology, I stained the culture slides and rinsed them under the tap. . . . My slides contained dividing cells with countable chromosomes, something I had never seen in ordinary tumor-tissue sections. I knew nothing of chromosomes or of the recent cytogenetic advances that had corrected the human chromosome number from 48 to 46,[57] but I thought somebody might be interested. My inquiries ultimately led to David Hungerford, a graduate student at the Institute for Cancer Research, who was doing a thesis on human chromosomes and needed material. Our collaboration resulted: I cultured the cells, and he looked at them. Our first cases, of acute leukemia, were unrewarding. Then Dave spotted a small chromosome in cells from two male patients with chronic granulocytic leukemia (CGL). These

findings were published with caution (because the Edinburgh group had found no abnormality in CGL) and with the suggestion that the "minute" chromosome might be an altered Y. Subsequent cases . . . led Dave to assign the minute chromosome correctly to the larger pair of G-group autosomes, first numbered 21 and later changed, by convention, to no. 22. . . . The Edinburgh group graciously suggested the name "Philadelphia (Ph) chromosome."[58]

It was named Ph[1] with the expectation of more to follow, but, so far, there has been no Ph[2].

The same small chromosome was observed in additional cases[59] studied in their laboratory and by the group in Edinburgh.[60,61] Among the 12 patients examined by Nowell and Hungerford, the Ph[1] chromosome was absent in only 1 person. A satisfactory specimen was obtained from this patient only when she was in an acute crisis and her peripheral leukocytes were almost exclusively "micromyeloblasts."[62] The authors thought that "the apparent presence of this chromosome change from the outset of the disease, plus the consistent finding of the same abnormal chromosome in association with this one particular form of leukemia, strongly [suggested] that it is this change in the genetic apparatus which confers on these cells their neoplastic character."[62] Tough et al. (1961) added that it seemed that chromosome 21 had lost a portion of its longer arm.[61] Also in 1961, Sandberg and colleagues reported that chemotherapy did not seem to enhance chromosomal anomalies; on the contrary, the chromosome counts of two patients with aneuploid leukemias in remission reverted, during therapy, to the normal 46.[63]

For more than a decade the Ph[1] was the only chromosome marker correlated with a specific neoplastic disease. It opened the door to the cytogenetic study of hematologic disorders.[64] Although the Ph[1] was initially believed to be a chromosome 21 (the chromosome associated with Down's syndrome), studies by Prieto et al. (1970) revealed that it originated in a chromosome 22. By identifying in the cells of a patient with chronic myelogenous leukemia (CML) a marker G that later converted to the Ph[1] chromosome, they were able to localize the chromosome from which the Ph[1] originated.[65] The development of quinacrine mustard fluorescence analysis allowed Caspersson et al. (1970) to identify the abnormality accurately as a partial deletion of the long arm of 22. They also stated that "a translocation cannot be excluded with certainty."[66] Rowley, by using both quinacrine fluorescence and Giemsa staining techniques, was able to show that the missing material had been translocated to the distal end of the long arm of a number 9 chromosome.[67]

Patients who present with a history and findings compatible with the diagnosis of CGL but who lack the Ph[1] chromosome usually have atypical clinical features.[68] Ezdinli et al. (1970) studied 61 patients with "typical chronic myelocytic leukemia" and found Ph[1] chromosomes in 43 of them. Those who were Ph[1] negative had a higher median age and were usually male. The median duration of survival was 40 months for Ph[1]-positive patients but only 8 months for Ph[1]-negative patients.[69] Canellos (1977) found that less than 10 percent of persons with classic clinical and hematologic features of CGL lack the Ph[1] chromosome. He cited 18 months as the median duration of survival for the Ph[1]-negative group, as opposed to about 40 months for the Ph[1]-positive patients.[70] More recently, investigators using molecular genetic techniques have shown that the correct diagnosis in many of the patients who are Ph[1] negative is a myeloproliferative disorder rather than CML; this helps to explain their poorer prognosis.

Recently, it has been shown that intensive chemotherapy may render the bone marrow free of any detectable Ph[1]-positive metaphases. Unfortunately, Ph[1]-positive cells reappear in virtually all patients after treatment is discontinued.[71] Suppression of the Ph[1] chromosome has also been observed after prolonged therapy with interferon.

For many years the Philadelphia chromosome was considered to be a characteristic unique to CML. This abnormal chromosome is also found, however, in patients with acute lymphocytic leukemia (ALL) or acute myelogenous leukemia (AML). Dewald et al. stated that the final diagnosis of 180 patients with a 9;22 translocation was CGL for 172, ALL for 4, AML for 3, and an unclassifiable acute leukemia for 1.[72] The Ph[1] chromosome in patients who have ALL is discussed in chapter 8.

Trisomy 15

Except for the Ph[1] chromosome, trisomy 15 of murine leukemia has been the most consistent leukemic cytogenetic characteristic (in fact, a prerequisite) known. Stich published pioneering work in this field. It is a known fact that rats develop hepatoma after being fed 7,12-dimethylbenz[α]anthracene (DMBA), but mice seem to be resistant to this carcinogen when fed in the same manner. Stich gave newborn mice one or two subcutaneous injections of DMBA. Lymphosarcomas of the thymus started to develop after 9 weeks and affected about 50 percent of the mice at 4 months after DMBA. No mouse not injected developed a leukemia. The thymus and spleen of the leukemic mice enlarged, and the lymph nodes in 52 of 55 showed marked enlargement. According to Stich, cytogenetic study "shows a correlation between altered chromosome complements and the occurrence of neoplastic cells, and the preference of one particular chromosome number."[73] His work showed that the leukemic cells invariably exhibited 41 chromosomes instead of the diploid 40. Subsequently, with banding techniques, other investigators identified this extra chromosome as number 15.[74]

Mutation

In 1953, Nordling wrote that "the cancerous cell contains not one but a number of mutated genes. . . . Statistics . . . show that the frequency of carcinoma increases according to the sixth exponent of age in males."[75] He believed that the high incidence of "internal neoplasms" during childhood is explained by the high frequency of cell division in the fetal stage. Nordling had examined the age-specific mortality from cancer of all sites in published statistics of the United States, the United Kingdom, France, and Norway.[76] According to Ashley (1969), Nordling had postulated that "carcinogenesis might depend on a series of mutations and that the clinical manifestation was dependent on the cumulative effect of this series of mutations."[76]

Knudson (1971) reviewed 48 cases of retinoblastoma seen at the University of Texas M. D. Anderson Cancer Center between 1944 and 1969. He formulated a two-step mutation hypothesis that has been accepted as an important advance in genetic etiology.[77] Hsu (1987) summarized Knudson's theory:

> A target gene must be mutated in both homologous chromosomes to change a normal cell into a malignant cell. The probability of having mutational events occurring in both genes simultaneously is obviously negligible. Thus, two genetic changes, in two steps, are the minimum requirements. However, if one mutation is inherited as a constitutional defect, then only one mutational event is needed to accomplish the malignant conversion.[78]

Knudson's hypothesis is supported by current cytogenetic and molecular biologic data and also has been broadened to other tumors; cases of leukemia may have a similar origin.

Since, basically, genes control cell growth and regulate cell proliferation, it is reasonable to look for abnormalities (because of mutation, reciprocal translocation, multiplicity, etc.) in the way genes function as a fundamental or contributing cause of cancer. By the late 1980, researchers had identified nearly 50 oncogenes associated with malignant disease.[79] Yarbro clarified:

> An initial mutation in the genome of a cell may confer a survival advantage on that cell. If one of the progeny of that cell is hit by a second mutation that confers an additional survival advantage, this new clone grows even more vigorously. A sequence of such events leads to the selection of a clone with the characteristics of a neoplasm; it also allows that clone to progress through ever greater stages of virulence characterized by invasion, metastatic spread, drug resistance, and other characteristics that ultimately lead to the death of the host. The genes in which these mutations take place have been called oncogenes or growth control genes.[2]

bcr-abl Hybrid Gene

Oncogenes may be positioned at the breakpoints of certain chromosomal irregularities that have been related to malignancies. The cellular *abl* (c-*abl*) oncogene was studied by Collins et al. (1984). In three Ph[1]-positive cell lines, they demonstrated the presence of a c-*abl*-related messenger RNA (mRNA) that is absent from cells of non-CML origin. The expression of this mRNA increases during blast crisis. As they wrote: "Malignancy is probably a multistage process involving a series of genetic changes rather than a single mutational event. One such genetic change in the pathogenesis of CML appears to be the acquisition of the Ph[1]."[80]

Other investigators have found a similar-sized *abl*-related RNA transcript in the leukemic cells of five of six patients with Ph[1]-positive CML, but none in those with Ph[1]-negative CML.[81] The oncogene *abl*, which resides on chromosome 9, is translocated to chromosome 22 as part of the Philadelphia chromosome.[81] In fact, as stated by Kloetzer et al. (1985), "two oncogenes are exchanged in this translocation (de Klein et al., 1982[82]), the c-*abl* gene on chromosome 9 (Heisterkamp et al., 1982[83]) and the c-*sis* gene on chromosome 22 (Dalla Favera et al., 1982[84])."[85] Sequences from the c-*abl* locus on chromosome 9 are fused to sequences in a breakpoint cluster region (*bcr*) on chromosome 22,[86] and this becomes the main consequence of the translocation.[82]

In the CML-derived cell line K562, Ph[1] is accompanied by a structurally altered c-*abl* protein (P210) with in vitro tyrosine kinase activity not detected with the normal c-*abl* protein (P145).[87,88] Konopka and colleagues thought that, "the altered P210 c-*abl* protein is strongly implicated in the pathogenesis of CML."[88]

Maxwell and associates (1987) examined leukocytes from patients in the blast crisis stage of CML for expression of P210[bcr-abl] tyrosine kinase activity. Phosphorylation of P210[bcr-abl] was observed in blast cells from four Ph[1]-positive CML patients in crisis. This activity was detected regardless of whether the blast cells were myeloid, lymphoid, or undifferentiated. No such activity was detected in leukocytes from four patients with Ph[1]-negative CML in blast crisis, from five patients with AML, or in the myelocytic cell line HL-60.[89]

Research is under way to develop methods for assessing the *bcr-abl* protein levels in tissues and fluids of patients with Ph[1]-positive leukemias and also to observe any changes in these levels during various stages of disease and during remission. Elevated levels of anti-*bcr*-reactive protein have been detected in CML patient sera; these levels revert to the normal range when patients achieve remissions. It may prove possible to monitor patients to aid in clinical decisions regarding starting and stopping medication and for prognosis.

Experience has shown that about one third of patients with Ph-negative CML have characteristics and prognoses similar to those of persons with Ph-positive disease.[90] Molecular analyses of 23 persons with Ph-negative CML revealed that in 11 the *bcr* showed rearrangement, indicating that this abnormal event occurred without the apparent documentation of the Ph chromosome. Patients who had the *bcr* rearrangement responded excellently to α-interferon-based regimens (seven of seven, 100 percent) and exhibited characteristics similar to those of patients with Ph-positive disease.[91] It seems that the diagnosis of CML may depend on the demonstration of the *bcr-abl* rearrangement whether the patient is Ph positive or negative, and, therefore, no one who lacks *bcr-abl* has CML.

SECONDARY LEUKEMIA

In 1978 three publications described the occurrence of CGL in a renal transplant recipient.[92–94] The patients were all men (ages 20, 22, and 40 years) who had received azathioprine and prednisone for prolonged periods of 3 to 4 years. Azathioprine is capable of a direct effect (e.g., chromosomal breakage) on the chromosome complement of marrow cells.[92] Thus, this drug in itself may be the culprit. Of course, a person with a suppressed immune system is in a very vulnerable state and at great risk of succumbing to infections or cancer. Cases of leukemia (usually acute myelogenous) after treatment for Hodgkin's disease have also been reported.[95]

Kingston et al. (1987) identified 151 children who had developed more than one primary neoplasm at intervals longer than 1 year. Fifty children (33 percent) had been treated with either single- or multiple-agent chemotherapy, which included an alkylating agent in 38 patients. Forty-five children had received a combination of chemotherapy and radiotherapy and, of these, 10 developed leukemia as their second tumor. Of the 19 secondary leukemias, 16 occurred in patients treated after 1970.[96]

THREE

Early Research in Cancer Chemotherapy at the National Cancer Institute

*Creative people are very unskeptical,
for to them everything is conceivable.*

FUNDING

In 1954, officials at the National Cancer Institute (NCI) were asked by members of Congress to consider a comprehensive program for research in cancer chemotherapy. It was decided that basic research would be advanced more by independent efforts of research groups around the country than by studies conducted by the federal government. Also, the NCI would ensure cooperation among the dispersed research groups by sponsoring seminars and symposia and by publishing an informal newsletter. Congress awarded almost $1 million in grants to a few prominent research institutions and medical schools for studies in cancer chemotherapy.[1]

Cancer Chemotherapy National Service Center (CCNSC)

In 1955, the CCNSC was established as the staff organization responsible for coordinating and operating the entire research enterprise, and four small committees were created to represent the main program areas: Chemistry and Drug Development, Drug Evaluation, Endocrinology, and Clinical Studies. Dr. Kenneth Endicott was chief of the CCNSC and was successful in attracting scientists of very high caliber. Congressional interest continued, and funds were available to expand and support all areas of endeavor.[1] One of these was the journal *Cancer Chemotherapy Reports*, whose inaugural issue appeared in January 1959.

Endicott was a pathologist who jokingly referred to himself as a failure in his chosen field. According to him, the administrative appointments he received were merely maneuvers calculated to keep him out of the way; they were positions where he couldn't do too much damage. He was subsequently named director of the NCI, was very skillful in dealing with Congress, and somehow managed to surround himself with ingenious, creative co-workers.

Zubrod

C. Gordon Zubrod arrived at the NCI in 1954 as Clinical Director and later (1961) became Scientific Director. In recent years,

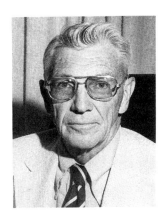

he has been referred to as the "Father of Chemotherapy" because, as DeVita wrote; "one person meant the difference between success and oblivion for the cancer drug development program and cancer chemotherapy and that person was, in fact, Gordon Zubrod. In addition to helping implement new concepts for the treatment of cancer with drugs, he bore the brunt of the criticism in and out of the National Institutes of Health [NIH][2]

Criticism at that time was widespread and vocal: "as much energy was expended in the scientific community

C. Gordon Zubrod

to stop cancer drug development as was exerted to get it off the ground."[2] Cancer had always been perceived as a localized disorder amenable to surgery or irradiation if diagnosed early. The medical community only slowly began to see it as a systemic illness; physicians had to be convinced, over time, to accept chemotherapy. Today we realize that sometimes cancer is a systemic disease almost from the onset, with clinically unrecognized micrometastases.[3]

During that early period, however, investigators at the NCI

made important contributions and became forerunners in the studies that led to the first drug cures of cancer.[4] Before the advent of chemotherapy, surgery and irradiation cured about one third of the patients with cancer. After the addition of chemotherapy, the cure rate rose to 41 percent (1979).[3,5]

Farber

During the 1950s, Sidney Farber was a prominent figure in medical politics as well as in cancer medicine. He had influence with Congress and stressed the need for clinical facilities at the NIH. In 1953, a campus hospital was opened.[6] Farber later showed the politicians photographs of a child with leukemia before and after treatment. He was accompanied and supported by Mary Lasker and Cornelius Rhoads, and this presentation resulted in a $1 million appropriation for leukemia research (1953).[4]

Burchenal

Before 1955, when several young clinicians arrived at the NIH, the laboratory facilities, which had developed from the original

U.S. Public Health Service, housed investigators who were involved primarily in basic science research. After 1955 the focus changed. Joseph Burchenal of the Sloan-Kettering Institute for Cancer Research was one reason for the difference. He went frequently to Bethesda to help the young physicians. He was a pediatric oncologist, a senior consultant, and an associate of many scientists who were powerful in the established medical community. He can best be described, however, as a very gracious, generous person who came and worked for days

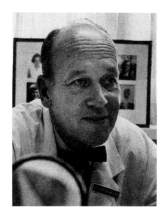

Joseph H. Burchenal

at a time to help solve problems, to review research and protocols, and to support the inexperienced neophytes in innumerable ways. He nominated them for membership in the foremost medical societies and was instrumental in making the NIH acceptable to academia.

Congressional allocations increased; in 1970 the budget of the NCI was $180 million, and by 1977 it had reached $815 million.[7] According to Shorter: "Congress thought it was financing revolutionary cancer therapies. What it did was to help finance with cancer money the revolution in biotechnology. For one thing, about half of the cancer institute's budget would be spent on basic research rather than on applied studies."[6] Out of this research came most of the biochemistry of recombinant DNA technology.[6]

PIONEERS

Goldin

Many outstanding investigators who devoted their lives to research of chemotherapeutic agents became prominent in the 1950s. One of them, Abraham Goldin, joined the NCI in 1949 and soon developed an active group of associates who became known for painstaking experimental drug research. They investigated many antileukemic compounds in mice and showed that drug effectiveness is influenced by various factors, such as (1) the time at which treatment is initiated, (2) the spacing of treatments, (3) the number of treatments, (4) administration of a metabolite, (5) the concentration of leukemic inoculum, and (6) the age and weight of the mice.[8–12]

Goldin often spoke of "therapeutic index," a principle that goes back to Ehrlich. According to Lane, "the thesis of selective toxicity was enunciated by Ehrlich: Successful chemotherapeutic agents must have high affinity for and high lethal effects on the parasitic cells, contrasting with their affinity for and effects on the cells of the host."[13] Lane continues: "In contrast with microbial invaders, parasitic cancer cells are derived from the cells of the host. . . . Consequently, the drugs used in chemotherapy have a narrow therapeutic index, and similar toxic effects are inflicted upon both neoplastic and normal cells."[13]

Citrovorum factor (CF) was first described by Sauberlich and Baumann of the University of Wisconsin in 1948,[14] and Goldin and colleagues studied it, particularly the time frame in which it was administered.[15,16] In 1953, they wrote that "an effective procedure for tumor treatment would be one in which an ordinarily lethal dose of aminopterin is administered alone but is followed by a delayed treatment with a massive dose of CF. This would permit the aminopterin to selectively damage the tumor, while the added CF is made available to the host before extensive damage to the host has occurred."[15]

Systematic screening procedures designed to uncover chemotherapeutic agents for use against cancer were instituted in 1944.[17] At the inception of the CCNSC, agents were screened against three animal tumor systems, leukemia L1210, sarcoma 180, and mammary adenocarcinoma 755. Later, for a wider selection that would predict activity of agents for clinical use, some 20 animal tumor systems were used routinely.[17] In the CCNSC program the total number of tumors used was over 100.[18] A retrospective analysis was conducted after 10 years of experience with the screening program of the CCNSC, and it was determined that L1210 plus Walker carcinosarcoma 256 (intramuscular) could have identified almost all of the agents as active.[18]

Law

The *L* in L1210 is for Lloyd Law, who discovered L1210 and who was considered by Zubrod to be the NCI's greatest biologist.[4] In 1949, Law was studying the growth inhibition of transplantable L1210 ALL in mice after administering aminopterin,[19] and he is still at the NCI in 1990. L1210 became a superb quantitative tool for studying antileukemia drugs,[4] enabling Law to evaluate systematically the effects of many agents on transplanted mouse tumors. He is an authority on the resistance of leukemic cells to antineoplastic agents. In 1956 he wrote that "the problem of resistance in neoplastic cells, as in microorganisms, will remain a most important perpetual threat to the successful use of therapeutic agents."[20] His publications cover a wide range of topics, including thymus structure and function, tumor immunotherapy, the immunologic surveillance mechanism, and

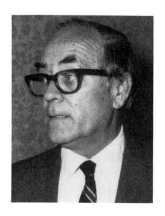

Lloyd W. Law

immunosuppressive agents, as well as mechanisms of resistance to many drugs.

Holland

James Holland left the NCI around 1954 to become Chief of Medicine A at Roswell Park Memorial Institute, but his group

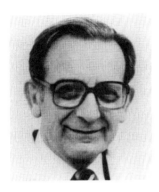

cooperated with Zubrod and colleagues at the NCI in the early clinical trials of leukemia. Holland's publications, like those of Law, encompass many areas of cancer medicine and have appeared in the most prestigious medical journals over the past four decades. He studied the effects of many drugs, including disodium ethylenediaminetetraacetate (EDTA) in hypercalcemic patients,[21] urethane and azaserine in those with multiple myeloma,[22] folic acid antagonists,[23] and vincristine in persons with advanced cancer.[24] In 1974, he and Emil Frei edited *Cancer Medicine*, a two-volume text, and wrote chapters entitled "Principles of Management of Cancer Patients" and "Selected New Developments." In more recent years, Holland has been Professor and Chairman of the Department of Neoplastic Diseases at Mt. Sinai School of Medicine, and his publications in the 1980s reflect his long experience and his broad perspective, as well as his common sense ("Breaking the Cure Barrier,"[25] "Randomized Trials in Rare Tumors,"[26] "Adjuvant Chemotherapy of Osteosarcoma: No Runs, No Hits, Two Men Left on Base"[27]).

James F. Holland

Frei

Emil Frei III arrived at the NCI as a senior investigator in 1955, was promoted to Chief of the Medicine Branch 2 years later, and also served as head of the chemotherapy service. He became Zubrod's good and reliable right arm.

In 1965, he went to M. D. Anderson Cancer Center and was an outstanding Associate Director for Clinical Research until 1972.

Since then he has been Physician in Chief at the Dana Farber Cancer Institute and Professor of Medicine at Harvard.

He received the Lasker award in 1972, was designated as the Man of the Year by the American Cancer Society in 1981, and was honored with the Kettering Prize from the General Motors Cancer Research Foundation in 1983. He has written extensively on many aspects of cancer, especially chemotherapeutic agents.

Stock and Phillips

During the period of Joseph Burchenal's tenure at the Sloan-Kettering Institute, accomplishments in the Division of Experimental Chemotherapy were outstanding. The names of Chester Stock (biochemist) and Fred Phillips (father of preclinical toxicology) are prominent because of their many important contributions to the body of information on chemotherapy. Stock began working with nitrogen mustards and continued with folic acid analogs, 6-mercaptopurine, and many others. In the 1970s he published detailed results of experiments with amygdalin. Phillips also worked extensively with nitrogen mustards, aminopterin, thioguanine, and subsequent agents; his work on the pharmacology of mitomycin C was meticulous.

Rall and Loo

David Rall became head of experimental therapeutics at the NCI in the late 1950s, and T. L. Loo was an outstanding member of his team. Loo later transferred to M. D. Anderson Cancer Center and gained a wide reputation for his work on the pharmacology of numerous antitumor agents.

Many other pioneers who arrived at the NCI in the 1950s and 1960s contributed to the origin and development of fundamental concepts that led to subsequent successes and cures benefiting today's patients.

FOUR

Chemotherapy with Single Agents

"Hope" is the thing with feathers
That perches in the soul
And sings the tune without the words
And never stops—at all.

Emily Dickinson (1830–1886), " 'Hope' is the thing with feathers"

It could be said that the earliest documentation of therapy for malignant disease occurred in the first century A.D., when Dioscorides wrote of colchicine. He stated that *Colchicum lingulatum* was useful for tumors if they had not spread.[1,2] Farber considered that Paracelsus (1493–1541) should be credited with having initiated the field of chemotherapy because he spoke of a specific chemical within the cell "wherewith to drive out the venoms of a specific disease."[3] John Hunter, the great surgeon of the 1700s, noted that castration resulted in progressive atrophy of the prostate.[4] This observation was used in subsequent attempts to cure prostate enlargement by orchiectomy. Later, in the 1940s, the concept led to a widely accepted therapy for prostate cancer.

Lissauer (1865) demonstrated that potassium arsenite (Fowler's solution) had antineoplastic activity.[1,5] In 1896, Sir George Beatson of Glasgow introduced bilateral oophorectomy and administered thyroid extract to treat advanced cancer of the breast.[4,6]

Ehrlich reported his discovery of the first alkylating agent in 1898.[7] In studies on the constitution, distribution, and pharmacologic action of various chemicals, he described the pathologic effects of ethylenimine on the cellular components of certain organs.[8,9] It was nearly 50 years later, however, before this observation was applied to the treatment of neoplastic disease. In 1964, Haddow recalled "the prophetic view of Paul Ehrlich, as long ago as the turn of the century, that of all the many chemical agents he had ever examined, ethylenimine struck him as unique, in its potentiality to induce irreversible change in the properties of protoplasm—an

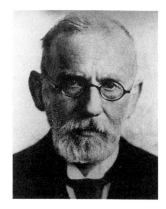

Paul Ehrlich

observation so remarkable as to establish him as the true pioneer in this field as in so many others."[10] Ehrlich also coined the term *chemotherapy* and defined it as the treatment of a systemic parasitic disease with a chemical of known constitution.[7] Around the turn of the century, Ehrlich worked on cancer but was not at all optimistic about the result. In fact, one who worked with him related that the area of the laboratory devoted to cancer research had a sign over it: "Abandon hope all ye who enter here."[7]

In 1902, Pusey tried radiotherapy for various disorders. Among those mentioned in his publication were a case of Hodgkin's disease in a 4-year-old boy in whom x-rays caused regression of large lymph nodes in the neck and a case of leukemia in a 50-year-old woman with an enormous spleen and a white-cell count of 300,000. She was given irradiation over the spleen with no effect whatsoever. The exposures were not carried to the point of producing visible changes on the skin.[11] Subsequently, irradiation to the spleen became a common therapy for leukemia because it usually reduced the size of that organ, lowered the leukocyte count, and relieved symptoms. The duration of control, however, was rarely longer than 6 months, and repeated courses of treatment were necessary.[12] Total body x-irradiation ("spray irradiation") was introduced in the early 1930s but gained little favor.[13] In more recent years, whole-body irradiation has been used as therapy and also for immunosuppression.

In 1909, Osler wrote that recovery from leukemia occasionally occurred but that the great majority of cases proved fatal within 2 to 3 years. The important general treatment, he wrote, included fresh air, good diet, and abstention from mental worry and care. Certain remedies had an influence on the disease, and of these he considered arsenic, given in large doses, to be the best. The curious remissions that occurred made evaluation of therapy hazardous.[14]

According to William Woglom, whom Shimkin described as a scholar of cancer:[15]

> Those who have not been trained in chemistry or medicine . . . may not realize how difficult the problem of cancer treatment really is. It is almost—not quite, but almost—as hard as finding some agent that will dissolve away the left ear, say, yet leave the right ear unharmed: So slight is the difference between the cancer cell and its normal ancestor.[16]

Woglom had reviewed 600 papers relating to immunity to transplantable tumors and stated in 1929, "Nothing may be hoped for at present in respect to a successful therapy [for cancer] from this direction."[17]

ALKYLATING AGENTS

Nitrogen Mustard

The military use of mustard gas (sulfur mustard) began with World War I, and information on toxicity was acquired from observing victims and from autopsies. Krumbhaar and Krumbhaar (1919) wrote that mustard gas exerts a direct toxic action on the bone marrow that depletes circulating leukocytes and also inhibits the regeneration process.[18] Meyer (1887) had earlier noted the poisonous and vesicant effects of sulfur mustard on rabbits.[9,19]

In 1943, during World War II, the Allied forces had established a base at Bari Harbor in Italy. German planes raided the harbor, and a ship loaded with 100 tons of mustard gas and with explosive munitions was hit. Not counting blast casualties, there were 617 mustard casualties, 83 of them deaths. Early deaths were from shock, systemic effects of mustard burns, and pneumonitis. The entire respiratory tract was often blistered from the vapor inhalation; pneumonia frequently ensued. Later, toxic injuries to liver, kidney, and hematopoietic systems took their toll. When victims died of infections, leukopenia and atrophy of lymph nodes and spleen were often noted.[20]

Pharmacologic studies of sulfur mustard in experimental animals were undertaken in 1941 by the U.S. Army. Louis Goodman and Alfred Gilman in the Department of Pharmacology at Yale University were asked to study the chemistry of nitrogen mustard (an analog of sulfur mustard) as part of the Army project. They noted destruction of bone marrow and lymph nodes and asked Dr. Tom Dougherty in the Department of Anatomy for a suitable animal tumor model. He supplied a mouse with a large lymphosarcoma.[21] Nitrogen mustard caused the tumor to disappear. As Dougherty recalled:

> I cannot remember exactly how many doses we gave, but in any case, the tumor completely regressed to such an extent that we could no longer palpate it. . . . We stopped treating the animal and the regression remained for a period of a month or more before a very slight growth began to appear. We then treated the animal again and the regression occurred again, although it was not as complete as the first time. In any case, the tumor did decrease and finally began to grow again, at which time further treatment brought about no inhibition of growth.[22]

They had experienced the same disappointment that subsequent investigators have faced—the malignant cells became resistant to the drug.

In 1963, Gilman recalled the circumstances surrounding the first injection of nitrogen mustard in a human (1942). Inasmuch as dramatic results had been achieved in mice that had lymphomas, it was decided to use the drug on an x-ray-resistant patient in the terminal stages of lymphosarcoma. He had tumor masses involving the axilla, mediastinum, face, and submental regions; chewing and swallowing were almost impossible, and a tracheotomy set was kept close at hand. A full therapeutic dose of the nitrogen mustard was selected with "unwarranted confidence," and the patient was treated daily for 10 days.

> Within 48 hours after initiation of therapy, a softening of the tumor masses was detected. It soon became obvious that this

was not wishful thinking. By the fourth day of treatment, obstructive signs and symptoms were relieved and by the tenth day, when the series of injections was terminated, cervical masses were no longer palpable and a few days later the axillary masses had completely receded. The excitement generated by the dramatic remission was heightened by the fact that the total white blood cell count remained above 5,000 per cu. mm. during the ten days of treatment, predominantly, aging granulocytes. We were not unaware of the shift to the right in the granular series because the hematologic observations were in the capable hands of Jean Dougherty. Its true portent soon became very apparent. In an inexorable manner the geriatric granulocytes slowly died off and between the third and fourth week following the initiation of therapy the total white blood cell count hovered around 200 cells per cu. mm. There was an attending severe thrombocytopenia.[22]

The first reports of clinical trials of nitrogen mustard in the treatment of hematologic diseases were published in 1946.[23,24] Goodman and colleagues reported that its use for 67 patients with Hodgkin's disease, lymphosarcoma, or leukemia achieved salutary results in the first two and in those with chronic leukemia. Responses were varied in patients with acute and subacute leukemia.[23] Jacobson et al. used nitrogen mustard to treat 59 patients with Hodgkin's disease, lymphosarcoma, sympathoblastoma, multiple myeloma, myelogenous leukemia, polycythemia rubra, or lymphatic leukemia. Those with acute leukemia or multiple myeloma failed to respond, and the most encouraging results were largely confined to persons with Hodgkin's disease.[24]

Cornelius Rhoads' contribution in this area was substantial.[25,26] In a lecture in 1946 he reviewed the early research with nitrogen mustard and called it a "little mouse" that the mountain had brought forth. As he said: "This is the first mouse of this type which has ever been produced, and it might very well become the parent of a great race of new chemical compounds, one of which might be more useful than x-ray. If one chooses to be really fanciful and imagines an organization able and willing to exploit this new principle, it would develop something of importance."[26]

Something important *was* exploited and developed. The nitrogen mustards became valuable aids for palliating leukemias and lymphomas and are still used in curative combinations for Hodgkin's disease. Malignant diseases of the blood-forming organs or of lymphoid tissues are the foremost targets in chemotherapy "simply because they are amenable to little else and by nature they represent in fact metastatic growths, being widely disseminated . . . at their inception."[26]

Busulfan

In an effort to enhance the therapeutic efficacy of the nitrogen mustards, Sir Alexander Haddow and the group at Chester Beatty Research Institute in London (1948) developed other compounds with an ability to alkylate. One compound in particular, busulfan (Myleran), showed an intense inhibitory effect on hematopoiesis at a low dose of the drug. In rats, the main depressing action was on circulating neutrophils; therefore, a small group of patients with CML was studied in a clinical trial.[27,28] Galton (1953) gave Myleran orally to 19 such patients and found that it depressed myelopoiesis without seriously affecting other hematopoietic elements. All patients responded initially to treatment, but 9 relapsed within 6 months. Eight patients obtained remissions of 6 to 21 months. Thrombocytopenia was the only important side effect, but Galton believed that it was unlikely to be serious if large doses were avoided and if treatment were withheld when the platelet count was below 100,000 per cu mm.[29]

In 1977, Tartaglia explained:

> Since 1951, . . . busulfan (Myleran) has been the mainstay of treatment [of CGL]. It is easy to administer and readily produces a remission of peripheral blood abnormalities. . . . [It may be] continued for several months until the peripheral blood becomes normal. The spleen will gradually shrink and frequently becomes impalpable. During this period, the serum uric acid level must be monitored and any increase must be controlled with drugs such as allopurinol.
>
> When the peripheral blood becomes normal, . . . busulfan may be terminated and begun anew when the white blood count again begins to rise, or the patient may be placed on a small maintenance dose to keep the white cell count within normal range.
>
> . . . this remission does not extend to the bone marrow or

the Philadelphia chromosome, and the overall median survival time is only about 36 months. . . .

Eighty to 85 per cent of patients with chronic granulocytic leukemia undergo a . . . "blast crisis" . . . of the leukemia. The anemia becomes worse, thrombocytopenia occurs and splenic size increases. The percentage of myeloblasts in the peripheral blood begins to rise, and the marrow shows increasing immaturity of the granulocytic series. Many new chromosomal abnormalities become superimposed on the Philadelphia chromosome. This phase . . . is rarely responsive to therapy, and death usually ensues within a few months.[30]

Chlorambucil

Another drug developed at the Chester Beatty Institute was chlorambucil, a water-soluble aromatic nitrogen mustard. Among 62 treated patients, Galton et al. (1955) reported that 20 achieved striking remissions—4 with Hodgkin's disease, 7 with lymphocytic lymphoma, 4 with chronic lymphocytic leukemia (CLL), and 5 with follicular lymphoma.[31]

At present, chlorambucil is used as palliative treatment in cases of CLL and malignant lymphoma. It is not curative.

Cyclophosphamide

Cyclophosphamide (Endoxan, Cytoxan) was developed by Arnold, Bourseaux, and Brock at Asta-Werke Pharmaceuticals in Germany. It was described in the literature in 1958,[32,33] although a symposium the previous year had included accounts of first experiments with the drug.[34] Herbert Arnold and Friedrich Bourseaux were chemists, whereas Norbert Brock is an oncologic pharmacologist; Hilmar Wilmanns, a clinical oncologist, also participated. They believed that, despite the drug's inactivity in vitro, the malignant tumors contained phosphatases and phosphoramidases that would convert cyclophosphamide into an active metabolite.[1] Later, it was shown that this conversion takes place in the liver by means of microsomal enzymes. The resulting product is the first "alkylating metabolite."[35]

Cyclophosphamide shows a significantly greater selectivity against many kinds of tumor cells than other cytotoxic agents of the nitrogen mustard series. "The wider margin of safety . . . is mainly due to its reduced general and organotropic toxicity; this has been shown by its less pronounced leucotoxicity, which in addition is more readily reversible."[35]

In 1959, Coggins and colleagues reported the treatment of 95 patients with the new cyclophosphamide. They achieved short remissions and some relief of symptoms in those with various types of carcinoma.[36] During 1960, the action of cyclophosphamide was discussed in five articles by different groups of authors.[37-41] One of these groups noted that platelet levels were not depressed: "The platelet-sparing

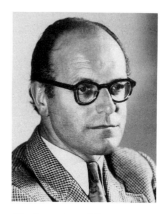

Herbert Arnold

effect appears to be a unique property of this drug."[39] Another commented that the absence of gastrointestinal symptoms from cyclophosphamide was a distinct advantage.[40] The most comprehensive publication (Hoogstraten et al., 1960) cited results of a trial by the Acute Leukemia Cooperative Group B. Ninety-seven patients (43 children, 54 adults) with advanced acute leukemia received cyclophosphamide on two oral dose schedules, 2 mg/kg/day and 10 mg/kg/week, and 82 patients were deemed evaluable. The overall remission rate was 11 percent. Although remissions were more frequent with the weekly dose schedule (15.2 percent) than with the daily schedule (6 percent), the difference was not statistically significant.[41]

Over the years Cytoxan has continued to be a very important chemotherapeutic agent. Although effective alone against susceptible malignancies, it is more frequently administered concurrently or sequentially with other antineoplastic drugs. It is used not only against lymphomas and leukemias, but also against multiple myeloma, carcinoma of the breast, adenocarcinoma of the ovary, retinoblastoma, and neuroblastoma.[42]

Ifosfamide

Synthesized by Arnold, Bourseaux, and Bekel of Asta-Werke Chemical Research Laboratories, a new alkylating agent, ifosfamide, was introduced at the Fifth International Congress of Chemotherapy in 1967 in Vienna.[43] Subsequently, ifosfamide underwent

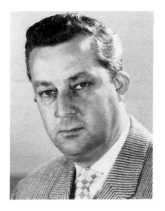

Friedrich Bourseaux

comprehensive pharmacologic testing and also in vivo trials in rats and mice. It is a derivative of cyclophosphamide but proved to be superior to cyclophosphamide against several animal tumors.[44] It was less toxic in animals, showing a wider margin of safety and a lower leukotoxic effect than other cytostatics. According to Brock, "Cumulation of the curative action is enhanced, whereas cumulation of the toxic action is reduced."[45] Because of increased reversibility of toxic effects, the intervals between administrations could be shortened, which meant higher total doses brought into action within shorter periods of time.[45]

Scheef of the Jankers Institute of Radiotherapy in Bonn spoke at the Seventh International Congress of Chemotherapy in Prague (1971) on his experience with ifosfamide. He had used the drug since 1969, treating 141 patients who had advanced malignancies, predominantly oat cell bronchiogenic carcinoma, ovarian carcinoma, and breast cancer. One hundred five persons who faced a life expectancy of 2 weeks to a few months before treatment were evaluable. These 105 patients received a total of 124 single massive doses; on 22 occasions the single doses were 90 mg/kg and on 6 occasions they were 150 mg/kg. Ifosfamide was injected intravenously (i.v.) over 3 minutes as a 5 to 10 percent aqueous solution. There were full remissions in 29 patients and partial remissions in 21; the treatment failed in 27; evaluations were not feasible in the remaining 28 persons. In addition, all patients received radiotherapy. Three died with severe hemorrhage originating in the urinary passages, including kidney tubules. This complication was subsequently prevented by good hydration, bladder instillation of a cysteine solution, administration of a saluretic drug, and alkalization of the urine, as hemorrhage occurred only with acid urine.[46]

In 1972, van Dyk and associates stated that experimental evidence had shown that definite cures of transplantable tumors could be achieved by one single dose of ifosfamide. They reported a clinical trial using single large doses for 37 patients with far-advanced metastatic disease. "As the curative effect in animals depends on concentration rather than on total dose administered, it seemed logical in clinical toxicity studies to determine the largest single dose that could safely be given to patients."[47] Their first 7 patients received 50 or 80 mg/kg every 2 weeks, repeated one to six times. The next 24 patients received 150 mg/kg, repeated monthly. Their therapy included bladder instillations of a cysteine solution and good hydration. Unfortunately, an unexpected, severe nephrotoxicity was encountered in this group, and the final cohort of 6 patients was given only 10 mg/kg for 5 days a week. In all 6, granular cylinders were found in the urine—evidence of tubular damage.[47]

Rodriguez and associates (1976), at M. D. Anderson, stated that ifosfamide produced hemorrhagic cystitis in 40 to 50 percent of the patients who received the drug in single high doses. As an alternative, i.v. infusions (over 1 to 2 hours) of 600 to 1200 mg/sq m/day for 5 days were given to 32 patients whose cancers were refractory to prior therapy. Of these patients, 11 had acute leukemia, 3 had malignant lymphoma, and 18 had various solid tumors. There was microscopic hematuria in 14 percent and gross hematuria in only 10 percent. Azotemia was not encountered. There was an antitumor effect in 7 of 27 evaluable persons.[48]

Because no sizable study had used ifosfamide for hematologic malignancies, this same group in Houston administered the agent to 27 patients who had acute leukemia and to 15 patients who had malignant lymphoma refractory to previous therapy. The basic dose was 1200 mg/sq m as a daily continuous infusion for 5 days; every 2 to 3 weeks the regimen was repeated. No responses occurred among 10 patients with AML, but 47 percent of those with ALL or acute undifferentiated leukemia responded. Seven of 15 persons with malignant lymphoma responded. No significant urinary tract toxicity occurred.[49] With the exception of the failures in patients with AML, these results were encouraging because disease in all patients had previously proved to be refractory to the most highly regarded agents available, and some of the patients had advanced disease that had progressed on other regimens.

During this same period, Brock and colleagues at Asta-Werke

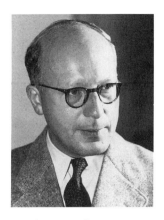

Norbert Brock

had been investigating the urotoxicity of oxazaphosphorine cytostatics.[50] They showed that the concomitant administration of sodium 2-mercaptoethane sulfonate (mesna) could also prevent the hemorrhagic cystitis.[51,52] Case et al. (Cancer and Leukemia Group B) recently (1988) cited results of a phase II trial of ifosfamide and mesna in previously treated patients with non-Hodgkin's lymphoma. Among 31 evaluable persons, 3 (10 percent) developed hemorrhagic cystitis.[53]

Ifosfamide-mesna is a highly effective combination that is administered as a single drug. It eliminates the problem of hemorrhagic cystitis and greatly expands the range of malignant conditions against which ifosfamide is useful. The combination is valuable against lymphoma, leukemia, and a wide variety of solid tumors.

In general, combination chemotherapy is superior to treatment with single agents. Norberg et al. in Sweden investigated ifosfamide combinations in the treatment of advanced bone marrow neoplasms. The authors used a near-maximal dose of ifosfamide and moderate doses of vinblastine, Adriamycin, or methotrexate. The side effects were consequently considered to be caused mainly by ifosfamide. A response to therapy was obtained in 8 of 15 patients. Of 2 patients with AML, one had no response and the second had a partial response. Side effects were mild considering the wasted state of the patients. Total-body baldness occurred in all persons receiving more than two courses of treatment. Mesna was given to protect the bladder and proved to be very successful.[54]

Evaluation of 49 adult patients with ALL in relapse who were given two dosage levels of teniposide in combination with ifosfamide was accomplished by Ryan and associates with the Southwest Oncology Group. They used two treatment regimens: 18 patients received teniposide (30 mg/sq m) on days 1 to 5 and ifosfamide (1,000 mg/sq m) by continuous i.v. infusion on days 1 to 5. When side effects were acceptable, the dose of teniposide was increased. Thirty-one patients received teniposide (50 mg/ sq m) on days 1 to 5 in addition to ifosfamide. Complete remissions were observed in 11 percent of those who received the lower-dose schedule and in 19 percent of those who received the higher dose. Hematologic toxicity occurred in most patients: 84 percent had white blood cell counts less than 1,000/μl during induction therapy, and 78 percent had platelet counts less than 50,000/μl. Hematuria was dose limiting in four persons.[55]

HORMONES

In 1941, Huggins and Hodges found that prostatic cancer is influenced by androgenic activity in the body. "With respect to serum enzymes, prostatic cancer is inhibited by decreasing androgenic hormonal function and activated by increasing the androgens."[56]

Dougherty and White (1943) wrote that the existence of a reciprocal relationship between the size of the adrenal cortex and the thymus had been known for some years.[57] In fact, Ingle had reported in 1938 that "the administration of large amounts of cortin causes marked involution of the thymus in the intact rat."[58] Deficient adrenal secretion results in hypertrophy of the thymus. As Dougherty and White related: "Recently, pure adrenotropic hormone has been prepared, making possible the study of effects of normal physiological stimulation of the adrenal cortex on the thymus. The paucity of data concerning the effects of adrenal cortical secretion on the mass of lymphoid tissue suggested careful studies of lymph nodes, spleens, and thymi."[57] They tested 41 mice, 12 of which acted as controls. Injecting pure pituitary adrenotropic hormone produced a decrease in weight of the inguinal, axillary, and mesenteric nodes and of the thymus. The spleen did not show a weight decrease.

At the suggestion of Dougherty and White, Dameshek (in 1943) treated two patients suffering from CLL with crude pituitary adrenotropic hormone extract daily for 2 weeks but, as no results ensued, further studies were not carried out.[59]

In 1949, Pearson and co-workers undertook a trial to determine whether the rate of growth of various types of neoplastic tissues in humans would be influenced by increasing adrenal cortical function. Seven patients (three with CLL and one each with lymphosarcoma, Hodgkin's disease, carcinoma of the prostate, and metastatic carcinoma of the breast) received adrenocorticotropic hormone (ACTH) and one patient (with CLL) received cortisone. They were given a total of 100 to 200 mg of the hormone daily for 18 to 30 days. The six patients with lymphomatous tumors showed a dramatic and progressive decrease in the size of enlarged lymph nodes and spleen, but the two patients with carcinoma showed no obvious change. None of the participants reached a complete clinical remission.[60]

At the First Clinical ACTH Conference in 1949, Farber related that ACTH therapy had brought about complete remission in a 6-year-old boy whose bone marrow had consisted of 98 percent blast forms.[61]

Rosenthal et al. (1951) used ACTH or cortisone to treat 42 persons with various diseases of leukocytic proliferation. Children with acute or subacute lymphocytic leukemia had a high immediate remission rate (69 percent). The remissions were, unfortunately, brief in most cases. Although the authors believed that treatment must be intensive and prolonged, they concluded that "certain cases of lymphosarcoma and chronic lymphocytic leukemia may be strikingly improved."[59]

After many similar hormonal compounds were tried, prednisone became the most widely accepted and has gained use in many of the combination chemotherapy protocols used today.

URETHANE

The Chester Beatty group, which was so prolific in the 1940s, also discovered the antitumor effects of urethane. In 1946, Haddow and Sexton found that urethane retarded the growth of spontaneous cancers in mice. When it was tried in humans, it induced a fall in the leukocyte count, prompting the researchers to test it in patients with leukemia.[62] That same year, they published an account of urethane action in 32 such persons. Results included a decrease in the white blood cell count to normal, a tendency for the differential count to approach a more normal pattern, shrinking of the spleen and enlarged lymph nodes, and a rise in hemoglobin. No permanent benefit was indicated because relapses occurred, but the palliative effect was "very great in many instances."[63]

ANTIMETABOLITES

Until the late 1940s, leukemia generally progressed in an inexorable manner, unchanged by any known treatment. Death came all too soon. At that time, however, the discovery of a drug effective against acute leukemia did much to change the prevailing attitude of distrust of chemotherapy.

Folic Acid Antagonists

For years it had been known that green leafy vegetables contained factors that were important in the formation of blood cells. One of these, *Lactobacillus casei* factor, was shown by Leuchtenberger et al. (1944) to be a strong inhibitor of tumor growth.[64] One year later, the same group observed complete regressions of spontaneous breast cancers in 38 of 89 mice treated with daily injections of *L. casei* factor.[65]

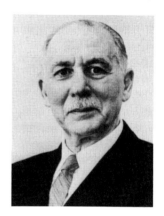

Sidney Farber

Later, it was recognized that pteroyltriglutamic acid, a contaminant in the extract, was the active agent.[66] That acid was an antimetabolite of folic acid.[1] A deficiency of folic acid, one of the B vitamins, deters hematopoiesis, and Heinle and Welch (1948)[67] and Farber (1949)[68] noted that folic acid accelerated the leukemic process.[1] Some of the folic acid analogs were even more potent as growth stimulators. At Lederle Laboratories, Dr. Yella Subbarow, who was studying various folic acid and folic acid antagonist compounds, supplied aminopterin for clinical study to Farber and colleagues at Boston Children's Hospital. They achieved temporary remissions in 10 of 16 children with acute leukemia.[69] The striking success of this trial became a motivating and energizing force for research in cancer chemotherapy.

In subsequent years, aminopterin has been replaced by methotrexate (amethopterin), which has the distinction of being the agent used in the first drug cure of cancer. Li and associates used methotrexate to treat a young woman who was terminally ill with choriocarcinoma. They began treatment in October 1955, and by February 1956 all evidence of disease was gone.[70]

Methotrexate was believed to be as effective as aminopterin and less toxic; it was reported to have a better therapeutic index in L1210 mouse leukemia.[71] Subsequently, it has been shown that aminopterin has at least five times the antifolic activity of methotrexate and thus potentially offers a much greater antileukemic effect.[72] The reputedly greater toxicity of aminopterin in comparison with methotrexate may have been the result of impurities in the former. When aminopterin (supplied by Lederle) was analyzed by Oliverio (1961) at the NCI, he found it to consist of 85 percent pure aminopterin, 8 percent folic acid, and 7 percent unidentified pteridines and unrelated compounds.[73] To our knowledge, trials using a purified aminopterin against acute leukemia have never been conducted, but they might prove very rewarding.

In ALL, methotrexate is used today for prophylaxis and treatment of meningeal leukemia and also as a component of combination maintenance therapy. It is used alone or in various combinations in the treatment of breast cancer, lung cancer, and epidermoid cancers of the head and neck. It also is indicated in the management of severe, recalcitrant psoriasis or rheumatoid arthritis.[42]

6-Mercaptopurine

This is one of the chemotherapeutic agents that, like 5-fluorouracil, resulted from biochemical reasoning aimed at antitumor effect.[1] It was evident by 1942 that folic acid (*L. casei* factor) and purine and thymine metabolism were intimately related. At that time efforts were initiated at Wellcome Research Laboratories in New York by George Hitchings and Gertrude Elion to prepare antimetabolites related to purines and pyrimidines, primarily for the insight a study might provide regarding details of nucleic acid metabolism.[74] Thioguanine was first prepared in 1948, but subsequent attempts to repeat the procedure met with failure and only the first batch was available for testing. Then, 6-mercaptopurine (6-MP, a purine antagonist for *L. casei*) was synthesized, and this process was more successful. Both drugs were submitted for testing as possible antitumor agents in 1951. The first trial of 6-MP produced a negative result, and thioguanine was very toxic; further experiments were necessary to determine a tolerated dose. Later, repeated experiments established 6-MP as a tumor inhibitor, and Law (1953) reported its activity against leukemia.[74] Law found that 6-MP inhibits cell growth of L1210 (ALL) in a "definite, regular, and reproducible manner."[75] "The observations of Clarke et al.[76] [1953] on the failure to grow transplants of tumors from animals [treated with 6-MP] and the discovery of regressions of sarcoma 180 subsequent to therapy indicated an unusual type of activity for this new antimetabolite."[74]

Burchenal and colleagues (1953) reported that 6-MP produced good clinical and hematologic remissions in 15 of 45 children who had acute leukemia; another 10 showed partial remissions. Adults suffering from acute leukemia occasionally achieved remissions with 6-MP, and in a few cases it produced temporary remissions in both early and late stages of CML. The most important toxic effect was bone marrow depression with the resultant leukopenia, anemia, thrombocytopenia, and bleeding.[77]

Mercaptopurine was used later in the well-known VAMP combination against ALL and, under the name Purinethol, is still of use in various combinations for initial remission induction and for maintenance therapy for ALL. Administration of Purinethol as a single agent is not justified.

Thioguanine is still used as a component of combination anticancer therapy for remission induction, consolidation, and maintenance against AML.[42]

Hitchings and Elion received the Nobel Prize for Medicine in 1988 in recognition of their work with a number of drugs, including 6-MP.

Arabinosylcytosine

Arabinose nucleosides were first isolated from the sponge *Cryptotethya crypta* by Bergmann and Feeney (1951),[78] and 4 years later Bergmann and Burke isolated the uracil arabinonucleoside from the same source.[79,80] Several of the arabinose nucleosides exhibit activity against tumors and viruses.[81] However, the most powerful cytotoxic agent is cytosine arabinoside (Ara-C), first synthesized chemically by Walwick and associates (1959) at the University of California at Berkeley.[82]

Chu and Fischer (1962) of Yale University experimented with murine lymphoblasts (L5178Y) and concluded that cytosine arabinoside inhibited the reproduction of leukemic cells by repressing the reduction of cytidylic acid to 2'-deoxycytidylic acid. Cytosine arabinoside prevents synthesis of DNA and cell reproduction.[83] In 1965, these same authors isolated a clone of L5178Y cells resistant to Ara-C and compared various properties of these resistant cells with those of the sensitive parental line. Chu and Fischer suggested that resistance to Ara-C is related to the inability of resistant cells to convert it to Ara-C monophosphate; they also believed that Ara-C nucleotides are incorporated into both DNA and RNA.[84,85] Cohen stated that the term *cytosine arabinoside* is incorrect as *arabinoside* defines a glycoside. In nucleosides, there is a glycosyl linkage, and the correct term is *arabinosylcytosine*.[85]

Evans et al. (1961), at the Upjohn Research Division in Kalamazoo, Michigan, demonstrated the activity of this new drug against recently transplanted and established sarcoma 180, Ehrlich carcinoma, and L1210 leukemia in mice.[86]

In the initial clinical trial of Ara-C, Talley and Vaitkevicius (1963) wrote that this substance is unique among available pyrimidine or purine antimetabolites in that both of its moieties, base and sugar, occur naturally: cytosine is a normal constituent of all living cells and arabinose is a sugar present in some foods. The drug induced objective, but temporary, decrease in some lesions in 2 of 10 treated persons with disseminated carcinomatosis. In doses of 3 to 50 mg/kg administered i.v. at various intervals, the drug induced definite megaloblastic changes in the marrow of all patients studied.[87]

In the first trial of cytosine arabinoside by Freireich and colleagues, the drug was given in a single i.v. injection, once daily, for 5 consecutive days separated by 9-day minimal treatment-free intervals. In eight patients there were one complete hematologic remission (12.5 percent), three inadequate trials, and four failures. While that trial was under way, Freireich et al. received the following additional information about Ara-C.

Schabel, Skipper, and colleagues had reported in 1965 that nondividing L1210 leukemic cells in vitro seem resistant to high levels of certain chemotherapy agents.[88] They later stated that "some antimetabolites, which on daily administration provide a significant increase in the life span of leukemic animals, were relatively ineffective in killing leukemia cells in vitro when the cells were in a nondividing state."[89] They found that arabinosylcytosine fit this category, and in 1967 they wrote: "Biologic and biochemical data suggest that arabinosylcytosine rather specifically blocks DNA synthesis. This mechanism of action infers [sic] that cell death results only when cells exposed to arabinosylcytosine are passing through the S-phase of their generation cycle."[89]

With this information in mind, Freireich et al. initiated a small study to test Ara-C by continuous i.v. infusion over a 5-day period, again separated by 9-day treatment-free intervals between courses of therapy. Of 14 patients with acute granulocytic leukemia, 6 (43 percent) achieved complete hematologic remissions, 2 achieved partial remissions, and 1 patient had significant improvement.[90]

In 1966, Ellison et al. reported the successful use of Ara-C against human leukemia.[91] They obtained 10 complete and 3 partial remissions in 48 adults with AML and 3 complete and 2 partial remissions in 9 adults with ALL. They administered the drug by continuous i.v. infusion.[92]

By 1968, Ellison's group had accumulated a larger cohort of patients treated with Ara-C and reported 16 percent remissions complete in all aspects, 3 percent complete except for hemoglobin level, and 6 percent partial remissions among 180 adults with AML. Twenty-four percent of 37 adults with ALL or unclassified leukemia had complete or partial remissions. They warned, however, that platelet transfusions should be available when Ara-C is used.[93]

Frei and colleagues of the Southwest Cancer Chemotherapy Study Group (1969) evaluated the effect of dose and schedule of Ara-C on bone marrow function in 88 patients with metastatic cancer of multiple types. Single doses of the drug produced no myelosuppression. Continuous infusion for 48 or 96 hours resulted in marrow depression along a steep dose-response curve. Continuous infusion of up to 1,200 mg/sq m over 24 hours increased the marrow depression, but further increase in dose did

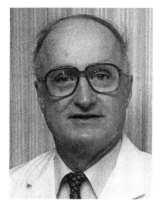

Emil Frei III

not cause more severe myelosuppression.[94] A decade later, when high-dose Ara-C was under consideration, this study became very useful because it was the only trial that had included research of single doses of various strengths.

Subsequently, the Southwest Oncology Group organized a prospective trial in which 185 adults with acute leukemia were randomly allocated to one of two cytarabine continuous intravenous infusion protocols: either 800 mg/sq m for 48 hours or 1,000 mg/ sq m for 120 hours. Courses were repeated for a minimum of three at 2-week intervals until remission or failure. Response rates were 20 percent and 38 percent, respectively.[95] These clinical studies demonstrated the importance of drug scheduling to achieve maximal effectiveness.

After many later trials, Ara-C became a very important drug for the treatment of AML. One of the significant changes in natural history that has occurred as a result of Ara-C therapy is the growing fraction of patients remaining alive and disease- and treatment-free for more than 5 years; most clinicians consider these persons cured of their disease.[96] The evidence to date suggests that Ara-C is primarily responsible for this change in natural history,[97] and, over the years, it has remained as the single most important agent available for treating AML.

Three of the first 15 patients with that diagnosis who were given Ara-C as a single agent at M. D. Anderson Cancer Center in 1969 and 1970 were still alive in September 1988. Before 1969, none of the M. D. Anderson Cancer Center patients with AML had survived 3 years.

During the 1970s and 1980s, the most commonly used regimens for AML combined Ara-C with an anthracycline antibiotic (daunorubicin or Adriamycin) and/or thioguanine. Vincristine and prednisone are also included in some schedules. Between 50 and 65 percent of adults with myeloblastic leukemia will respond to these combination protocols. The median duration of response is between 9 and 12 months. A cure fraction of 5 to 20 percent of the patients treated is an encouraging finding. Amsacrine (AMSA), etoposide, and high-dose Ara-C are newer therapies with recognized activity against acute leukemia. Brief accounts of the development and early trials for each of these are included in this chapter.

High-dose Ara-C

In the very early developmental work with Ara-C, as dose and schedule were being elaborated, Frei et al. (1969) administered Ara-C at a high dose (1,000 to 4,200 mg/sq m) as a single, rapid injection. This treatment was administered at 2-week intervals to 51 patients who had metastatic cancers of various types. The investigators noted no bone marrow toxicity, but also no antitumor effect.[94]

During the late 1970s, researchers suggested that the resistance of malignant cells to Ara-C might be due to certain biochemical processes that, in some cases, could be reversed by increasing the Ara-C dosage. Studies with malignant cells in vitro showed that resistance to Ara-C could be overcome by a "10–100 fold increase in Ara-C concentration above that effective against 'Ara-C sensitive' neoplasms."[98] Clinicians were eager to test this theory because, although the existing chemotherapy for acute adult leukemias was resulting in a high percentage of complete remissions, these remissions were frequently of short duration and the relapse rate was high.

In 1979, Rudnick et al. treated 13 patients whose leukemia was refractory to conventional treatment with 1.0 to 7.5 g of Ara-C per sq m over 29 drug cycles. Five patients were septic and terminally ill when treatment began. The regimen was well tolerated. One patient had a complete remission and three had partial remissions.[99]

Also in 1979, Karanes and associates reported treating 21 adults with acute nonlymphocytic leukemia (ANLL) in relapse with Ara-C (3 g/sq m every 12 hours by 2-hour infusion for 4, 8, or 12 doses). The dose was selected on the basis of the trial conducted by the Southwest Cancer Chemotherapy Study Group in 1969.[94] Six of 9 patients who received 12 doses had complete remissions and 1 had a partial remission. No remission was attained by 2 patients who received 4 doses. Three of 10 persons receiving 8 doses had complete remissions.[100]

In a large series, Herzig et al. (1983) used high-dose Ara-C to treat 57 patients who had refractory acute leukemia. They reported that the maximum tolerated regimen was 3 g/sq m every 12 hours for 6 days. Extending the duration of treatment to 8 days resulted in excessive diarrhea and skin erythema with bullae. Increasing the dose to 4.5 g/sq m every 12 hours for 6 days produced cerebellar toxicity. Among 37 evaluable patients who had AML, 70 percent responded, with 51 percent achieving complete remissions.[101]

Based on observations indicating synergy between sequential high-dose Ara-C and asparaginase, Capizzi and associates (1984) treated 32 patients who had acute leukemia (truly refractory in only 4). Patients were given 3-hour i.v. infusions of Ara-C (3 g/sq m) at 12-hour intervals for four doses, followed by asparaginase (6,000 IU/sq m) at hour 42. Among patients with ANLL, complete remissions were attained by 9 of 13 with no antecedent hematologic disorder and by 6 of 9 with an antecedent disorder. Three of 10 who had advanced ALL also achieved complete remissions.[98]

Preisler and co-workers (1984) with the Leukemia Intergroup Study reported the following results of high-dose cytosine arabinoside treatment for 110 persons who had ANLL: in 32 (29 percent), there was complete remission; in 43 (39 percent), induction failure was attributed to resistant disease; and in 35 (32 percent), treatment failed for "other" reasons.[102]

Keating et al. (1985) tried a variety of schedules for high-dose Ara-C in a study designed to investigate the relationship between intracellular levels of Ara-C triphosphate (Ara-CTP) and response. Shortening the time between doses to maintain a high intracellular Ara-CTP level did not increase complete remission rates.[103]

High-dose Ara-C has definitely improved response rates and median survival times of patients with AML. Various dosing schedules are still being evaluated.

L-ASPARAGINASE

Asparagine is a naturally occurring amino acid that was first characterized in 1806 by Vauquelin and Robiquet.[104] The enzyme,

L-asparaginase, was discovered by Lang (1904);[105] Clementi (1922)[106] showed that the guinea pig carries the enzyme in its blood.[1] It was not until 1953 that Kidd reported that

> transplanted lymphomas of two kinds regularly regressed following repeated injections of normal guinea pig serum intraperitoneally into mice carrying them, the animals meanwhile remaining lively and devoid of signs of illness or wasting. The lymphomas of untreated controls, by contrast, usually grew progressively and killed their hosts within 20–30 days, and the same was true of the growth of other mice given repeated injections of horse or rabbit serum.[107]

Broome (1961) found that "the L-asparaginase activity of guinea pig serum is responsible for the anti-lymphoma effect."[108]

When Old and colleagues (1963) examined the sera of many South American rodents for levels of L-asparaginase activity, they found that the agouti serum showed much greater activity than that of the guinea pig. In the latter, the highest value found was 169 units/ml of L-asparaginase, whereas the values in agoutis ranged as high as 720 units. The authors also found that the same quantitative relationship existed between leukemia inhibition and L-asparaginase activity, whatever the source.[109] This same research group treated three dogs that had advanced lymphosarcoma with L-asparaginase. All responded with marked lymph node regression and dramatic improvement in general condition without evidence of toxicity. This experiment showed that primary tumors were sensitive to this new agent; its effect was not limited to transplantable tumors in laboratory rodents.[110]

Dolowy et al. (1966) stated that certain lines of lymphoma cells require L-asparagine. Their work suggested the hypothesis that L-asparaginase can deplete the available L-asparagine in the body of mice below that required by tumor cells without seriously harming the host. They confirmed tumor regression in mice after administration of guinea pig serum and of bacterial L-asparaginase. They decided to try the experimental material on an 8-year-old boy in frank relapse after a 3-year battle with acute lymphoblastic leukemia that had failed to respond to therapy (prednisone, 6-MP, methotrexate, cyclophosphamide, vincristine, and irradiation to the central nervous system and right testis). Intravenous infusion of L-asparaginase caused marked hemolysis within 4 hours; 10 hemorrhagic bowel movements occurred during infusion. The boy was given blood transfusions but died of pulmonary hemorrhage 10 days after treatment. During the week after therapy, his lymphoblasts decreased from 76 to 14 percent, and both the liver and a tumorous testicle decreased in size.[111]

In 1967, two groups published data about patients treated with L-asparaginase. Hill et al. wrote that therapy for three patients with ALL resulted in measurable improvement in two with advanced disease; the third patient showed a striking response to a large dosage, with rapid necrosis of lymph node masses and clearing of leukemic infiltrates. Also, acute and chronic granulocytic leukemia were shown to be asparagine dependent.[112] Physicians at Sloan-Kettering Institute used L-asparaginase to treat seven patients who had leukemia and two persons with lymphosarcoma. They reported significant therapeutic alterations in four of those with acute lymphoblastic leukemia and in one with acute myeloblastic leukemia. Four patients did not respond.[113]

These were the early demonstrations of the effectiveness of this enzyme in humans. It has continued to be part of the induction strategy in regimens for ALL in both children and adults.

Today, it is believed that the malignant cells in some patients who have acute leukemia, particularly lymphocytic, are dependent on asparagine for survival; normal cells, however, are able to synthesize asparagine and thus are affected less by the rapid depletion produced by treatment with the enzyme asparaginase.[42]

L-Asparaginase was in short supply for the early clinical trials. It was very expensive and, on one occasion, physicians from the NCI went to Dallas to join with Hill in making a plea for funds from a wealthy Texas oilman. He was not inclined to contribute, but a pharmaceutical company did offer assistance.

NATURAL PRODUCTS

Vincristine

Alkaloids are organic substances found in many plants. They are usually very bitter, and many are pharmacologically active (atropine, caffeine, morphine, quinine, nicotine).[104] The plant *Vinca rosea* Linn (periwinkle) is an everblooming sub-shrub that has enjoyed a popular reputation in folk medicine in many parts of the world.[114] Peckolt (1910)[115] described the use in Brazil of an infusion of its leaves to control hemorrhage and scurvy, to clean and heal chronic wounds, and to wash the mouth for toothache.[114] In Europe, it has been used to suppress the flow of milk.[114,116] In the West Indies, tea made from its leaves was used to treat diabetes and diabetic ulcer,[114,117] and in the Philippines, also, it has been used as an oral hypoglycemic agent.[114,118]

Noble, Beer, and Cutts were working at the Collip Medical Research Laboratory at the University of Western Ontario in 1949, studying various plant extracts used by primitive people, when they received leaves of the periwinkle, *Vinca rosea*, from the West Indies. They found it to have no effect on carbohydrate metabolism. However, 5 to 7 days after they injected a water solution of periwinkle into rats, the rats died of multiple abscesses. On culture, *Pseudomonas* was consistently found, but these organisms were not present in the extract. Apparently some natural barrier to infection was being depressed. Before death, the rats exhibited a rapidly falling white blood cell count, granulocytopenia, and depression of bone marrow.[117]

The periwinkle plants were grown as an annual in Canada and, although active extracts could be obtained, the yield was about one quarter that found in plants from the West Indies, where periwinkle grows wild and is a perennial. Investigation was limited, but whenever material was available its carcinostatic activity was studied. It showed definite activity against transplantable adenocarcinoma in mice and against a transplantable sarcoma in rats.[117]

Often, in research, groups in different parts of the world follow similar paths unknown to each other. Irving Johnson and other scientists at the Eli Lilly Company in Indianapolis had been screening plant extracts in a search for new oral antidiabetic agents. They were using animals and checking blood counts at intervals. It was brought to Johnson's attention that one group of normal animals developed low white blood cell counts after receiving an extract of *Vinca rosea* Linn. In 1957, during routine cancer screening, he and his colleagues found antileukemic activity against P1534 lymphocytic leukemia in mice.[119] They began preliminary testing on patients suffering from cancer and also provided the

Collip group with material so further clinical studies could be carried out in Canada.[120]

A crystalline alkaloid was isolated and named "vincaleukoblastine" (VLB) by the Canadian group. This substance, when injected into rats, depressed the bone marrow, leading to a severe granulocytopenia. In mice bearing the transplantable leukemias L1210, P1534, and AKr or Ehrlich ascites tumor, treatment with VLB effectively prolonged survival. Mice "cured" of AKr or P1534 were subsequently resistant to repeated challenges by the tumor.[120]

Hodes and colleagues stated that 20 patients had received VLB, and all had experienced a drop in the peripheral total leukocyte count, with granulocytes affected most. Hemoglobin, erythrocytes, and platelets were generally affected slightly or not at all. Toxic effects included anorexia, nausea, stomatitis, epilation, and marrow depression. Complete hematologic remission was achieved in patients with ALL or monocytic leukemia. When hematologic remission was not achieved, tumor cell infiltrates were decreased in size.[121]

It was later found that the crude extract of periwinkle had greater ability to prolong survival than did the purified VLB. The drug vincristine comes from the more active material.[122] Johnson and Eli Lilly deserve credit for assuming the cost and having the persistence to get vincristine on the American market. During screening at the NCI, using CCNSC guidelines, the drug was not effective against L1210 or other tumor systems available. Lilly, however, used many of their own animal tumors in extensive experiments and found excellent activity against P388 leukemia. Later, the NCI agreed to add this to their screening list.

Karon, Freireich, and Frei (1962) with the NCI used vincristine sulfate (supplied by Eli Lilly) in a clinical trial. Fifteen consecutive patients younger than 16 years of age who were known to be refractory to 6-MP and methotrexate were treated with vincristine; all had previously received corticosteroid therapy. Two children who were given a small starting dose died before the second dose could be given. The report is based on the remaining 13 patients (12 with ALL, 1 with AML). Eight of the 13 had active meningeal leukemia, which was treated successfully with intrathecal aminopterin given with citrovorum factor to protect the bone marrow. Vincristine therapy was not interrupted during this additional therapy. Nine of the 13 children (69 percent) achieved complete remissions according to all criteria. Two patients, however, received steroids during the treatment course. Therefore, the minimal estimate for complete remission rate would be 7 of 13, or 54 percent.[122]

These were excellent and very encouraging results. Nevertheless, Johnson told the investigators that members of the Board of Directors at Eli Lilly were apprehensive about marketing the drug because proceeds would never equal or surpass the cost to the company as vincristine seemed to be effective only against childhood leukemia. Facing such an unfortunate possibility, clinicians from the NCI went to Indianapolis and appealed to the Lilly board to produce the drug for humanitarian reasons—the lives of these little children were at stake. Representatives from two other cancer centers also addressed the board. Lilly did market vincristine (Oncovin), and other early studies were published.

Carbone et al. (1963) used vincristine in 40 patients with malignant neoplastic disease in an effort to define its toxicity, tolerated dose, and antitumor properties. They found that toxicity is dose related and that toxic manifestations occur primarily in the neuromuscular system and gastrointestinal tract. These effects are reversible and not cumulative. In 4 of 10 patients with Hodgkin's disease, tumors regressed completely and in 6 they regressed partially. The median duration of regression was 4 months. Of 7 persons with lymphosarcoma, 3 had complete and 1 had a partial tumor regression.[123]

Selawry and Frei (1964) related that 56 of 66 children (85 percent) with ALL attained complete remissions with vincristine and prednisone.[124]

In time, vincristine became a very important chemotherapeutic drug, useful not only for acute leukemias, but also, in combination with other oncolytic agents, for Hodgkin's disease, non-Hodgkin's malignant lymphomas, rhabdomyosarcoma, neuroblastoma, and Wilms' tumor.

Daunomycin

In 1963, research workers in France and Italy independently isolated an antibiotic from cultures of *Streptomyces coeruleo-*

rubidus and *Streptomyces peucetius*, respectively.[1,125-27] The Italian team, from Farmitalia Research Laboratories in Milan, named the compound *daunomycin*, and DiMarco et al. (1964) first reported that it had significant antitumor activity.[128,129] In France, the drug was called *rubidomycin* (DuBost et al., 1964),[130] and it was subsequently shown to have physicochemical and biologic properties identical with those of daunomycin.[125]

Clinical trials have demonstrated that the drug can induce remissions in both acute lymphoblastic and acute myeloblastic leukemia.[125] Jacquillat and colleagues (1966) used rubidomycin for 5 days to treat 10 children suffering from advanced acute lymphoblastic leukemia resistant to usual antileukemic drugs. Among the 6 patients in whom the effects of the compound could be adequately evaluated, 4 achieved complete and 2 achieved partial remissions, all within a remarkably short time.[131]

Howard and Tan (1967) gave an account of combined daunomycin and prednisone induction in patients with acute leukemia. Seven of eight untreated and six of nine previously treated patients, most of whom had acute lymphoblastic leukemia, achieved complete or good partial remissions.[132] The following year, Holton and associates treated 39 children who had drug-refractory acute leukemia with daunomycin. Seven experienced remissions, and 4 of these 7 had received prednisone concurrently.[133] This suggested that the combination might be very effective for patients who had relapsed after conventional therapy. Therefore, as a joint effort of the Southwest Cancer Chemotherapy Study Group, 67 children with acute leukemia who had relapsed one or more times were treated with daunomycin and prednisone. Sixty had ALL and seven had AML. In the former group, 39 attained complete and 10 attained partial bone marrow remissions. Of the latter group, 1 had a complete and 1 had a partial remission.[134]

Adriamycin

Closely related to daunomycin, Adriamycin is also an anthracycline antibiotic that was isolated from a mutant of *S. peucetius*[135] in 1967 in the Farmitalia Laboratories.[136] DiMarco et al. (1969) reported testing for antitumor activity against ascitic and solid tumors. The survival time of treated animals was considerably increased, but chronic toxicity had not yet been tested.[137]

In the early clinical evaluation trials, Bonadonna and associates (1970) treated 155 patients (34 children, 121 adults) with Adriamycin between September 1968 and December 1969. The patients had solid tumors or various forms of leukemia. Ninety-four had received prior chemotherapy, irradiation, or both. Toxic manifestations included alopecia (in approximately 87 percent of the patients who received an adequate drug course), bone marrow depression (78 percent), oral ulcers (76 percent), gastrointestinal upsets (32 percent), and fever (12 percent). Irreversible bone marrow aplasia occurred in 11 of 15 persons who died during treatment with Adriamycin. The authors stated that, if Adriamycin is stopped promptly at the time of initial redness of the oral mucosa, bone marrow depression, although sometimes severe, is transitory. Four patients with acute leukemia achieved complete clinical and hematologic remissions, and two achieved partial remissions. In all 4 of the patients who had CML, the peripheral leukocyte count fell promptly and hepato- and splenomegaly regressed; 2 achieved complete remissions. The response, however, was short-lived and, unless patients were given maintenance therapy with other drugs, it never exceeded 5 weeks.[136]

In a 1975 review of Adriamycin, Carter stated that the drug has a broad spectrum of activity over many types of cancer, including malignant lymphomas and acute leukemias. He added that the toxic effects are dose related, predictable, and reversible. Cardiac toxicity causes the greatest problem in long-term treatment.[138]

In 1974, McCredie and associates at M. D. Anderson Cancer Center used sequential Adriamycin-Ara-C (A-OAP) for remission induction in adults aged 15 to 75 years who had acute leukemia. Thirty-three received Adriamycin followed on day 5 by Ara-C for 5 days as a continuous i.v. infusion, plus vincristine on day 1 and prednisone on days 1 to 5. A second course was started on day 19 and included appropriate dose adjustment, depending on bone marrow cellularity and blast cell count. Of 27 patients able to finish an adequate trial of therapy, 85 percent achieved a complete remission.[139]

For many years, Adriamycin has maintained prominence among cancer chemotherapeutic agents. It is useful against disseminated neoplastic conditions such as ALL; AML; Wilms' tumor; neuroblastoma; soft tissue and bone sarcomas; breast, ovarian, bladder, thyroid, gastric, and small cell bronchiogenic carcinomas; and both Hodgkin and non-Hodgkin lymphomas.[42]

AMSA

In 1933, Mellanby wrote:

When mammalian cancer tissue is treated with acriflavine [an acridine dye] for two hours at 37°C., it loses its power to take up oxygen while retaining its glycolytic action on sugar. The intensity of the action depends on the strength of the acriflavine solution; a 1 in 5,000 or stronger solution reduces the oxygen uptake 50 per cent or more and prevents all subsequent growth even if there is plenty of sugar present for the tissue to get its energy.[140]

Since then, many acridine congeners have been investigated as possible antitumor products.[141] Cain and Atwell (1974), in New Zealand, during "the course of a study of the structure-antitumor relationships in a series of bis-quaternary salts, . . . discovered a new agent which showed excellent activity in L1210 screening systems."[142]

The new agent was an acridine derivative, and the authors assessed three related compounds. Amsacrine (AMSA) was selected for clinical trial because it was not only effective against L1210 but also had been examined in the B16 malignant melanoma and P388 leukemia assays and produced long-term survivors in both.

In 1978, Gormley and associates studied the mechanisms by which AMSA exerts its selective toxicity, particularly its interaction with DNA. In its DNA binding it seemed similar to other acridines, and they believed that the cytotoxic effects probably resulted from a modification of DNA function.[143] Researchers in 1984, however, showed that the mammalian enzyme DNA topoisomerase II may be the primary cytotoxic target of AMSA.[144,145]

Animal studies revealed that the principal toxicity of AMSA was directed at the hematopoietic system (anemia, leukopenia, thrombocytopenia), although gastrointestinal side effects (nausea, vomiting, diarrhea) also occurred.[146] The first clinical trials were reported in 1978. Legha and colleagues at M. D. Anderson Cancer

Center treated 26 patients with doses ranging from 4 to 50 mg/sq m injected i.v. daily for 3 consecutive days and repeated at 3-week intervals. Bone marrow toxicity was dose limiting but was rapidly reversible. Responses were observed in 2 patients with adenocarcinoma of the lung and 1 each with melanoma and AML.[146]

Because bone marrow was the primary target of AMSA toxicity, there was immediate interest in evaluating its use against acute leukemia. Legha and associates (1980) treated 62 adults who had refractory acute leukemia with a total intravenous dose of 150 to 1,320 mg/sq m administered over 3 to 14 days. Fifty-six patients received an adequate trial and, of these, 13 achieved complete remissions and 6 achieved partial remissions. Complete remissions were achieved in 9 of 39 persons who were refractory to cytarabine and anthracyclines, indicating a lack of cross-resistance. The principal adverse effect was severe myelosuppression, which led to frequent infections during the therapy period.[147]

By 1982, Legha and associates had assessed AMSA in 109 adults (102 evaluable) who had acute leukemia that had previously been treated. They concluded that the optimum dose for remission induction is 120 mg/sq m/day for 5 days. Complete remissions were achieved in 28 percent of the patients with AML and in one patient with ALL; these persons were maintained on AMSA, 30 to 40 mg/sq m/day for 5 days repeated at 4-week intervals. The median duration of remission was 12 weeks, and responders survived significantly longer (27 weeks versus 8 weeks).[148]

Subsequently, AMSA has been used in combination with Ara-C,[149,150] Ara-C and 6-thioguanine,[151] and with Ara-C, vincristine, and prednisone (AMSA-OAP)[152] for induction and consolidation therapy.

It has been observed that patients with Auer-rod-positive acute leukemia respond better to AMSA than those who have the Auer-rod-negative type. Also, the response rate seems to be related to the quantity of previous treatment received by the patient.[153]

The activity of AMSA alone is comparable to that of the anthracycline antibiotics; however, the myocardial toxicity seen with the latter is rarely observed with AMSA.[154]

AMSA has proven to be a frontline drug, producing excellent results for patients with acute leukemia. It is available all over Europe but has not been released by the Food and Drug Administration (FDA) in the United States. Pharmaceutical companies are reluctant to embark on the expensive testing required for FDA approval when prospects indicate that the drug will have a relatively limited market. Recently, M. D. Anderson Cancer Center obtained a supply of AMSA for a specific study.

Etoposide

Podophyllin is a resin that has been used as a caustic topical application for certain papillomas. It is made from the dried rhizome and roots of the *Podophyllum peltatum* plant, commonly known as the May apple. In 1942, Kaplan wrote that treatment with this substance produced cures of condylomata acuminata,[155] and it is still in use today for that purpose. The active ingredient in podophyllin is podophyllotoxin,[156,157] which is a spindle poison with effects similar to those of colchicine. It arrests mitosis in metaphase.[157,158]

Greenspan et al. (1950) injected alpha-peltatin, beta-peltatin, and podophyllotoxin subcutaneously into mice bearing five types of transplanted tumors: acute stem cell leukemia, a metastasizing lymphosarcoma, a local lymphosarcoma, a mammary adenocarcinoma, and a melanoma. About 1,000 animals were used. A single injection of each agent induced extensive damage to all types of tumors, and metastases responded like the main tumor mass. No tumor, however, regressed completely. The substances delayed the rise in the number of stem cells in the peripheral blood of mice with leukemia.[159]

Subsequently, several cytotoxic podophyllum compounds were introduced, and Vaitkevicius and Reed (1966) reported clinical studies with two of them, SP-I and SP-G; results were inconclusive.[160]

During the 1960s, the research division of Sandoz Ltd. (Basel) developed a derivative, teniposide (VM-26), that had a high cytostatic activity in cell cultures. It inhibited entry of cells into mitosis or destroyed cells preparing for mitosis; a biochemical effect was the inhibition of thymidine uptake.[157]

In 1973, Dombernowsky and Nissen reported on the antileukemic activity of another podophyllotoxin derivative, etoposide (VP-16-213), a topoisomerase II-reactive agent like AMSA. Dombernowsky and Nissen found "a very high antitumour activity against L1210 ascites tumour, with divided treatment or treatment once daily every fourth day being the best schedules." Testing in mice showed up to 100 percent long-term survivors on the optimal schedules.[161]

Significant antileukemic activity for etoposide was demonstrated initially by Mathé and colleagues. In a study by the European Organization for Research on the Treatment of Cancer (EORTC), complete remissions were achieved by four of eight patients with either acute monocytic or acute myelomonocytic leukemia.[162]

In an early report of these two compounds (teniposide and etoposide) tested in childhood cancer, Rivera et al. (1975), from the St. Jude Children's Research Hospital, evaluated the drugs in 39 children who had not responded to the customary chemotherapeutic agents. Although none of the 10 patients with solid tumors responded, definite clinical benefit was obtained by 9 of 29 children with acute leukemia. The epipodophyllotoxins were well tolerated, although side effects included nausea, vomiting, diarrhea, fever, alopecia, leukopenia, and thrombocytopenia.[163]

Radice and colleagues (1979) accomplished therapeutic trials with both etoposide and teniposide for patients with solid tumors as well as those with lymphomas or leukemias. They reported that the objective response rate to etoposide was 25 percent for patients with AML and 41 percent for the subgroup with acute myelomonocytic leukemia. Surprisingly, neither etoposide nor teniposide showed significant activity against ALL (response rates of 7 percent and 14 percent, respectively).[164]

In a phase II study, the Children's Cancer Study Group (1979) evaluated the antitumor activity and toxicity of etoposide in 126 patients with childhood cancers. The medication showed significant activity against acute myelomonocytic leukemia, less activity against AML, and minimal activity against ALL. The major toxicity was neutropenia.[165]

Also in 1979, Rivera and colleagues treated 45 children with a combination of prednisone, vincristine, and teniposide. All had advanced ALL in marrow relapse and had not responded to previous therapy with prednisone, vincristine, and other traditional agents. Forty-two of 45 patients completed the 4- to 6-week regimen; 13 achieved complete remissions, 7 showed an oncolytic response, and 22 had no response. Remissions were attained in some children who had undergone as many as five hematologic relapses.[166] The following year, Rivera and his group at St. Jude's reported that combinations of teniposide and Ara-C represented an alternative remission-induction therapy for persons in whom initial regimens were unsuccessful. Nine of 14 such children with ALL achieved complete remissions.[167]

In the early 1980s, many more clinical studies of teniposide and etoposide were reported, and in the late 1980s other uses for etoposide have been investigated. Blume and Forman (1987) reported on the use of high-dose busulfan and etoposide as a preparatory regimen for second bone marrow transplantations.[168] Also, Kushner et al. (1987) evaluated the effects of etoposide on normal human marrow cells and representative lymphoma-leukemia cell lines to assess the agent's use for ex vivo marrow purging. Doses of etoposide that cleanse marrow of lymphoma-leukemia cells spare hematopoietic and stromal progenitors, as was demonstrated in long-term marrow cultures. A differential sensitivity was therefore apparent, which supports a function for etoposide in marrow purging.[169]

Recently, the possibility that epipodophyllotoxin therapy may increase the likelihood of the development of secondary AML has been raised. Pui et al. (1989) projected a 5 percent incidence of secondary AML after 6 years of follow-up in the ALL trials at St. Jude's Children's Research Hospital between 1979 and 1988. They observed 733 children who had received treatment against ALL.[170,171] Etoposide and teniposide are relatively recent additions to the list of antileukemic compounds, and both can cause breaks in DNA strands.[170] For reasons yet unclear, T cell phenotype was the risk factor most closely associated with secondary AML in the St. Jude study. All of their patients with T cell leukemia had received epipodophyllotoxin therapy as a component of the intensive drug regimens used at that institution.[170]

Mitoxantrone

In 1979, Murdock and associates from the Medical Research Division of American Cyanamid Company reported on a new antitumor agent. It was synthesized as part of a focus on the anthraquinone and amino moieties of Adriamycin as especially likely areas for its known intercalative binding to DNA. Various systems were tested, and one anthracenedione "was found to give a modest but reproducible increase in life span in mice inoculated with either the L-1210 or P-388 leukemias."[172] This agent was then altered and modified in an effort to produce more effective compounds. When tested against P388 leukemia, derivative 40 compared favorably with other anticancer agents in clinical use (Adriamycin, cyclophosphamide, daunorubicin, methotrexate, 5-fluorouracil).[172] After completing this work, the authors found that Zee-Cheng and Cheng of the Midwest Research Institute in Kansas City, Missouri, had previously (1978) reported their independent synthesis and antitumor evaluation of the free base corresponding to derivative 40 and of 11 related anthraquinones.[173]

In 1983, Smith stated that American Cyanamid Company had synthesized a number of blue anthracenedione dyes in 1939 for use in the fiber industry. "In the middle 1970s the planar structure and DNA-intercalating ability of a few of these compounds suggested that they might be tested for possible biological use as interferon-inducers and immune-modulators."[174] One was found to have cytotoxic properties and, after a series of new compounds had been synthesized, mitoxantrone was the one selected for study as an anticancer agent.[174]

In 1974, Adamson proposed "that the cardiac toxicity in the daunomycin-adriamycin molecule resides in the daunosamine portion, allowing the molecule to be taken up by the cardiac muscle while the antitumor activity generally resides in the chromophore moiety."[175] According to Bergsagel, "Adamson suggested that the amino sugar at carbon atom 9 on the doxorubicin molecule was responsible for its cardiotoxicity but not for its antitumor effects. Mitoxantrone lacks this amino sugar."[176]

The configuration of mitoxantrone resembles that of Adriamycin, and animal testing showed corresponding or greater antitumor activity with less cardiotoxicity.[174] Although all of the details of the means by which mitoxantrone mediates its action have not been completely worked out, it is known that it inhibits DNA and RNA synthesis.

Most of the early practical knowledge of patient therapy came from studies of advanced breast cancer; only a few small trials involved leukemia. In a phase I trial of dosage, Vietti et al. (1981) reported that the dose required to achieve complete remission in children was much higher than the maximum dose tolerated by adults.[177]

In 1983, in a phase II trial at M. D. Anderson Cancer Center, mitoxantrone was administered to 41 adults who had refractory acute leukemia. The majority of these patients had suffered two or three relapses. The starting dose varied from 4 mg/sq m/day for 5 days to 10 or 12 mg/sq m/day for 5 days. Three patients had a complete response and 1 had a partial response. An antileukemia effect was more frequent at the higher doses, but so was death after treatment.[178]

The Lederle Cooperative Group (1985) reported a total of 70 evaluable patients treated for refractory and relapsed acute leukemia. The best results were obtained in patients with acute myeloblastic leukemia in first relapse. The responses achieved (9 of 22 or 41 percent) equaled or surpassed those of other agents in common use.[179]

Starling et al. (1985) reported a 33 percent response rate among 24 children given mitoxantrone for refractory acute leukemia. None of the patients developed any clinical signs of cardiotoxicity.[180]

Numerous other clinical studies have been published since these early efforts; the overall response rate of patients with refractory acute myeloblastic leukemia is about 33 percent. The experience with ALL and CML in blast crisis has not been as encouraging.[181] The dose-limiting toxicity is myelosuppression when mitoxantrone is given on a single-dose, every-3-week schedule and mucositis when it is given daily for 5 days. Median periods of remission have been short. During the past 3 or 4 years, reports of mitoxantrone in combination with other agents (cytosine arabinoside, etoposide) have appeared. Response rates of up to 50 percent have been reported, but the number of patients treated has been very small.[181]

The efficacy of mitoxantrone seems to approximate that of the anthracycline antibiotics; it can be useful in specific instances because it is not totally cross-resistant with Adriamycin.

PROCARBAZINE

This drug was developed during studies of methylhydrazine derivatives for possible use as monoamine oxidase inhibitors. Bollag and Grunberg (1963)[182] found that 1-methyl-2-benzylhydrazine had antitumor activity in several transplantable rodent tumors.[183] Because the compound had a relatively weak effect on tumors and was very toxic to the liver, its chemical structure was methodically altered;[184] procarbazine was one of the results. Procarbazine is an unusual agent whose action does not resemble that of other cytotoxic agents. It has a marked effect on the mitotic cycle of cell division,[185] and its means of action has been compared with the indirect effects of ionizing radiation.[186]

Used alone, procarbazine did not become an important member of the chemotherapy armamentarium for the leukemias or lymphomas. It developed significance, however, as part of the MOPP program (Mustargen, Oncovin, procarbazine, prednisone) for Hodgkin's disease. Since the early 1980s, physicians have been alerted to the occurrence of second primaries, especially AML, in patients previously treated for Hodgkin's disease. Chemotherapy, particularly MOPP, seems to be the major offender. Strong indirect evidence indicates that the culprit is procarbazine; experimentally, it is a potent carcinogen. Frei believes that high priority should be given to producing and using curative regimens that exclude procarbazine.[187]

METHYL-GAG

Methylglyoxal-bis(guanylhydrazone) (methyl-GAG) has undergone a revival during the past 10 years. Historically, it goes back to 1898, when it was synthesized by Thiele and Dralle[188] in Germany.[189] A series of articles in *Cancer Research* by Freedlander and French in 1958 focused the attention of cancer therapists on its possibilities. Those publications described antitumor activity in L1210 mouse leukemia and in adenocarcinoma-755-bearing rodents.[190–193]

The precise means by which methyl-GAG acts remain somewhat obscure, but certain features are known. It interferes with polyamine biosynthesis.[194,195] Biologically, it also acts as a mitochrondrial poison[195,196] and binds to DNA.[195,197] In 1961, Regelson and Holland used parenteral methyl-GAG to treat 14 patients suffering from advanced neoplastic disease and reported severe gastrointestinal ulceration and hypoglycemia. The latter proved to be refractory to glucose administration and was fatal for 3 persons.[198] Freireich and colleagues (1962), in a similar phase I study, reported complete remissions in 9 of 13 patients (69 percent) who had AML.[199] This was a spectacular result when one considers that the prevailing rate at that time was 13 percent.[200] When Carbone, Freireich, and colleagues in 1964 used methyl-GAG to treat 20 patients who had acute leukemia, they achieved 11 complete remissions, 2 partial remissions, and a median survival of 187 days for patients who responded.[200]

The side effects included not only fatal hypoglycemia but also extreme myelosuppression and severe cutaneous and gastrointestinal ulceration. Their virulent nature discouraged further clinical trials at that time. As Mihich wrote in 1963, "The enthusiasm elicited by the activity of the drug against acute myelocytic leukemia and other human tumors is somewhat tempered by the frequent occurrence of dramatic toxicity and, consequently, by the recognition of the extremely narrow range of selective therapeutic effectiveness."[201]

After about 15 years of neglect, methyl-GAG was retested on a weekly infusion schedule instead of a daily regimen by the Southwest Oncology Group, who reported reduced toxicity in a phase I trial.[195,202] In 1979, Knight et al. described the treatment of 109 patients who had advanced malignancies refractory to conventional therapy. All received weekly intravenous infusions of methyl-GAG, starting at 250 mg/sq m/week. This dose was increased to 500 mg after the first 12 patients evinced no toxic effects and no response. Dosage was increased by 100 mg/sq m/week in the absence of toxicity and was reduced by that amount if persons had moderate or severe side effects. Sixty-five evaluable patients achieved 2 complete and 9 partial remissions; tumors regressed in an additional 9, who were classified as improved. Sixty-seven of the 109 patients had no toxicity; others developed mucositis, nausea, and vomiting. "Responses were observed in a wide variety of solid tumors, particularly types known to be unresponsive to chemotherapy."[202]

That article revived interest in methyl-GAG, and by 1983 at least 50 trials had been completed or were in progress in the United States.[189] During the past 5 years, many studies of methyl-GAG in combination regimens have been reported. These protocols were used mainly to treat recurrent or refractory lymphoma, non-small-cell lung cancer, and esophageal cancer.

Although methyl-GAG is still available, it is not widely prescribed at present. It has proven to be less effective than some other agents and it has unpleasant, although tolerable, side effects.

CURATIVE CHEMOTHERAPY

Pinkel has considered the hypothesis that antileukemic drugs induce remission by cytotoxicity, but that cures are attained only by drugs that act on DNA.

> Prednisone, vincristine, and L-asparaginase, singly and in combination, act promptly to induce remission of ALL by interfering in protein synthesis, assembly, or integrity. However, they have not proven effective in maintaining remission so that their use is generally confined to remission induction. On the other hand, the drugs that are effective in continuing remission for long periods and in curing ALL act by altering DNA structure as well as inhibiting DNA synthesis. For example, methotrexate produces chromosomal breaks and sister chromatid exchange; . . . Cytosine arabinoside causes DNA chain termination resulting in double replication of DNA segments. . . . The purine analogs, alkylating agents, and epipodophyllotoxins cause DNA strand breaks.
> . . . acute leukemias are cured by drugs that alter genetics while not destroying the capacity for hematopoietic proliferation. Specifically, in cured ALL, the capacity to proliferate lymphoblasts with phenotypic characteristics of ALL, but not their neoplastic growth characteristics, is retained.[203]

Pinkel believes that curative leukemia chemotherapy "alters the lymphoid leukemia cell strain so that it loses its proliferative advantage or succumbs to normal control mechanisms."[203]

FIVE

Adjuvant, Maintenance, and Combination Chemotherapy

A new principle is an inexhaustible source of new views.

MARQUIS de VAUVENARGUES (1715–1747)

ADJUVANT AND MAINTENANCE THERAPY

In referring to chemotherapy, *adjuvant* is generally used to indicate auxiliary therapy given to patients in remission in the hope of extending the disease-free period. Commonly, however, *adjuvant* seems to be used more often in association with solid tumors, whereas one generally refers to *maintenance* chemotherapy in leukemia.

As mentioned previously, Furth and Kahn in 1937 showed that "a single malignant white blood cell is capable of producing the systemic disease—leukemia."[1] Furthermore, physicians are never sure whether their initial therapeutic approach has achieved a cure or if some subsequent therapy might help them reach the goal of total cancer cell kill.[2]

Between 1941 and 1951, Osgood and Seaman (1952) treated 163 patients who had chronic leukemia with total-body spray irradiation or radioactive phosphorus. They repeated the treatment at specified intervals while the patients' conditions were ideal and their disease was in remission. As they wrote: "We do not stop administration of digitalis because the patient is no longer in congestive heart failure. Why should we discontinue regular therapy for leukemia because the patient is at the time symptom free?"[3] In 1952, the mean survival time of the 163 patients was slightly over 4 years, and 73 of them were still living. In using adjuvant therapy, these physicians from the University of Oregon Medical School demonstrated an innovative approach, placing them well ahead of their contemporaries.

Farber and associates wrote in 1956 that

> until recently there were two schools of thought concerning the management of a patient once a remission had been induced. Intermittent therapy meant inducing a remission, then stopping treatment until relapse occurred, then starting treatment again and to repeat this cycle until no further improvement could be achieved. Smith and Bell (1950)[4] modified this method by following the bone marrow with weekly aspiration, and stopping therapy when the total nucleated count fell to 30,000. This technique has not found wide acceptance. Maintenance therapy after inducing a remission has been used by Farber (1948);[5] this method has been gradually adopted.[6]

Some examples of the early application of the adjuvant principle will be mentioned briefly. Although they do not pertain to leukemia, they were important background studies that set the stage for subsequent chemotherapy protocols. Farber and colleagues were pioneers in the adjuvant precept when they used radiation of the lung after surgically removing a Wilms' tumor.[7] An additional important milestone was reached when actinomycin was successfully used as surgical adjuvant chemotherapy for children with Wilms' tumor[2] (Farber et al.[6,8,9]).

In the hope of preventing metastases, Cruz et al. (1956) administered nitrogen mustard, beginning on the day of operation, to patients who had malignant tumors.[10] Shimkin and Moore (1958) described a prospective cooperative trial designed to study adjuvant chemotherapy accompanying the surgical treatment of cancer.[11] Unfortunately, some of these early studies of adjuvant chemotherapy failed to demonstrate a difference in survival of treated persons versus controls.[2]

By the early 1960s, trials of new chemotherapeutic agents against acute leukemia were usually limited to those persons who had already received and become refractory to drugs of proven value. Such patients have active acute leukemia, and it is often difficult to discern whether subsequent signs and symptoms are toxic effects from the therapy or manifestations of the leukemic process.

Therefore, a trial was designed to test the effectiveness of a drug in prolonging the duration of remission of acute leukemia. Patients were to be in a good state of health, and physicians would be able to evaluate more precisely the therapeutic effect and the toxic properties of the agent. Also, because disease was in remission, treatment would not be complicated by supportive measures such as transfusions or antibiotics.

6-MP Prolongs Remission

6-Mercaptopurine was selected as the active agent. Ninety-two patients under age 20 entered the study; 62 (67 percent) had complete or partial remission induced by corticosteroids. Patients in remission were randomly allocated to maintenance therapy with either 6-MP or placebo. The median duration of 6-MP-maintained complete remission was 33 weeks; the median for placebo was 9 weeks. A sequential experimental design permitted analysis of remission times while the trial was under way, and the study was stopped after the remission times of 21 pairs of patients (42 patients) had been analyzed. Overall survival of the two groups was not significantly different because patients receiving placebo were switched to 6-MP when they relapsed.[12] This study was important because it outlined a model for subsequent evaluation of other agents. The article reporting the trial has been cited frequently in biomathematic literature because of the innovative analysis procedure, which was developed primarily by Gehan.

Researchers soon learned that the biology of a patient with active acute leukemia is entirely different from that of a patient whose disease is in remission and that drugs that fail to induce remission may be very effective in maintaining remission. The model described was able to detect such agents. As one of the major problems in treating acute leukemia is the short duration of unmaintained remission, identifying agents that can improve remission maintenance is of prime significance.[13]

Cytokinetic Studies

Frei recalled that, "in the early 1960s, Dr. Howard E. Skipper and his associates initiated a series of studies addressed to the quantitative biology of leukemia in mice and its perturbation by chemotherapy.[14] These studies have had a profound impact on our understanding of, and approaches to, therapeutic research in the clinic."[15] Frei explained that Skipper's group found that, for a given treatment, the fractional reduction of tumor cells, not the absolute reduction, is the constant. This constant fractional kill is independent of tumor burden. Researchers determined that patients with clinically overt ALL have a body burden of leukemia cells in the range of a trillion (10^{12}).[16] It is assumed that curative

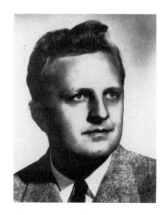

Howard E. Skipper

treatment requires the elimination of the entire burden. This is consistent with evidence from some of the transplanted mouse leukemias, in which a single cell is capable of ascending to overt disease. Complete remission-induction therapy destroys 1 kg of tumor and eliminates all clinical and laboratory evidence of leukemia. Although this involves a 99 percent or greater reduction in the number of leukemic cells, it is only the beginning of successful treatment, according to the first-order kinetic concept. Thus, just as much treatment is required to effect a 99 percent reduction from 10^{12} to 10^{10} cells (1 kg of tumor) as is required to effect a 99 percent reduction from 10^{6} to 10^{4} (less than 1 mg of tumor). Hence, continued treatment for a significant period after remission is essential to eradicate all leukemia cells.[15]

COMBINATION CHEMOTHERAPY

Skipper wrote in 1949, "It is generally agreed that urethane and the nitrogen mustard, HN^{2}, will consistently increase the survival time of mice and rats with certain strains of leukemia."[17] He experimented with 258 mice: 58 controls, 67 treated with HN^{2}, 68 treated with urethane, and 65 given a combination of HN^{2} + urethane. The average increase in life span over that of the controls was 80.5 percent for HN^{2} treatment, 44 percent for urethane treatment, and 150.4 percent for treatment with the combination. In mice, the two drugs did not seem to be synergistic with regard to toxicity. "Striking prolongations of survival time in [L1210] leukemic mice given various dosage levels of A-methopterin and 8-azaguanine simultaneously were obtained" by Law (1952).[18] "The objective of the work [of Skipper et al. (1954)] was to examine the feasibility of potentiating the antileukemic activity of a given agent by simultaneous administration of a second chemical which might be expected on the basis of biochemical knowledge to provide a sequential or a concurrent block in a series of biochemical events."[19]

According to Skipper et al.,[19] Potter (1951) introduced the term *sequential blocking* and defined it as "the action of two or more inhibitors, each of which acts on the same metabolic sequence but upon different enzymes within a limited portion of the sequence."[20] *Concurrent blocking* is an expression suggested by Elion et al. (1954)[21] to describe simultaneous blockade of two or more pathways concerned with the formation of the same end product.[19] Skipper's group found that

> the antileukemic activity of A-methopterin was potentiated by simultaneous administration of ethionine. This combination was synergistic with regard to antileukemic activity since ethionine alone does not significantly increase the life span of mice bearing L1210 or L4946 leukemia. In order to obtain maximum potentiation, the two drugs must be given at the same time. This suggests that blocking at one site and then later at another is not nearly so effective as simultaneous blocking two steps in a series of chemical events leading to a single end product.[19]

When 8-azaguanine was added, the triple combination was more effective than any dual combination of these agents.[19]

Before this time physicians were using single drugs on a continuous, interrupted, or sequential schedule, but Skipper's and other laboratory studies were soon followed by modest clinical trials of combined drug administration. Farber et al. (1956) found that laboratory experiments showed increased antineoplastic activity when folic acid antagonists and purine antagonists were given in combination.[6] Clarke et al. (1954)[22] showed a similar effect for the combination of 6-MP and azaserine[6] and reported that, for children with acute leukemia, "the combination of cortisone and either of the two commonly used antimetabolites has proved to be much more effective in the production of rapid improvement than cortisone or the antimetabolite when employed alone."[6]

First Cooperative Trial

In the mid-1950s, physicians at the NCI were treating only a limited number of patients, so the first group study was initiated in cooperation with Holland and associates at Roswell Park. This was the historic precedent for Cancer and Leukemia Group B. This first leukemia trial compared oral methotrexate plus 6-mercaptopurine given on a daily basis with the same two drugs given intermittently at 3-day intervals. The latter protocol was based on Dr. Goldin's animal work, which showed that intermittent doses of methotrexate produced a much better therapeutic index than continuous administration. The trial,[23] whose results were published in 1958, studied 84 children, 54 of whom were treated at the NCI. We believe that this report was the first publication describing a prospective randomized clinical trial of leukemia therapy, using the method introduced by Bradford Hill.[24]

Second Trial

At the time, however, the most noteworthy and widely publicized study was the second cooperative trial (1961).[25] It produced the first conclusive evidence that combination chemotherapy improved the complete remission rate of children with acute leukemia.[26] With 13 institutions collaborating, the study started in 1957 and continued for 3 years. Three programs for acute leukemia were compared: methotrexate followed by 6-MP, 6-MP followed by methotrexate, and both drugs given in combination. In children with ALL, the remission rate was 59 percent for the combination, 47 percent when 6-MP was the first drug, and 29 percent when methotrexate was administered first. Long-lasting remissions were more frequent in children who received the combination. In adults, the remission rate was 15 percent for the combination, 21 percent for 6-MP first, and 7 percent for methotrexate first. Survival longer than 5 months occurred more frequently in the combination group. Responsiveness to the second course of therapy was as good as that to the first course. Subsequently, when vincristine and prednisone were added, a complete remission rate of nearly 90 percent was achieved.[27,28] Blum et al. wrote that these studies "showed that selected agents can safely be used in combination at full or nearly full doses. This set the stage for the development of combinations of several drugs designed with curative intent, including the VAMP program for acute leukemia, the MOPP program for Hodgkin's disease, and others."[26]

Effects of Chemotherapy in Acute Leukemia

Also appearing in 1961, a report from researchers at the NCI attracted attention because the authors delineated for the first time several facts about chemotherapy and acute leukemia:

1. The proportion of patients who have ALL and achieve a complete remission with chemotherapy becomes progressively smaller as patient age increases. For those who have AML, however, the response does not differ according to age.
2. Patients who have ALL and are 19 years old or less survive the longest.
3. Patients who show some hematologic response to chemotherapy survive much longer than those in whom no such response is demonstrated.
4. This increase in survival time can be attributed directly to the time on effective chemotherapy.
5. A patient's response to the first course of chemotherapy has no value in predicting the chance of responding to a subsequent course of therapy.[29]

VAMP

By 1961, it was apparent to Zubrod and his colleagues that some minor inroads had been achieved in the battle against leukemia, and they were anxious to launch a major attack. The Acute Leukemia Task Force was formed to determine if, cooperatively, they could make an attempt at cure. Zubrod consulted with executives at IBM for advice on directing such an intensive, goal-oriented project. The Task Force included Holland, Frei, Freireich, Myron Karon, Farber, Skipper, Frank Schabel, Rall, Burchenal, Donald Pinkel, and many others.[30] Since 1955, Freireich had been working at the NCI studying the prevention of infection and the use of platelets to forestall or treat hemorrhage.

Vincristine and prednisone were known to produce a rapid induction of remission in ALL, with relatively little hematologic depression—but the remissions were very short. The members of the Task Force decided that four drugs would be used concomitantly along with intensive platelet replacement to prevent hemorrhage. Freireich, Karon, and Frei designed the VAMP regimen (1962) in an effort to eliminate residual leukemic cells and cure childhood ALL.[30]

They used a combination of vincristine, amethopterin (methotrexate), mercaptopurine, and prednisone (VAMP) administered simultaneously over a period of 10 days. Fourteen of 16 children achieved complete clinical and hematologic remissions. They were then given additional 10-day courses of therapy separated by 10-day or longer intervals of recovery from toxicity. After a median of five "consolidation" treatments, therapy was discontinued. The median duration of unmaintained remission was 5 months.[31,32]

The VAMP study was important not only because it was one of the early multiple-agent chemotherapy trials, but also because it was the first clinical trial to use early intensification treatment in an attempt to "cure" leukemia. The possibility of curing childhood acute leukemia became apparent from the VAMP results; approximately 10 percent of the participants were still disease-free at the last update (1984). Surprisingly, the results of the trial were published only in abstract form; the authors never took the time to write a complete paper because they were so anxious to undertake the next combination.[7]

Zubrod considered the cure of ALL to be the most important milestone in curative chemotherapy because the "Acute Leukemia Task Force provided the rational basis for curative chemotherapy by bringing together for one disease cell kinetics, pharmacology, supportive management toxicology, and clinical medicine."[7]

BIKE

The BIKE schedule used a combination of vincristine and prednisone to induce remission. Consolidation treatment consisted of a 5-day course of the maximum tolerated dose of methotrexate followed (after a 9-day or longer interval) by a 5-day course of 6-

MP. After another 9-day or longer interval, a single dose of cyclophosphamide was given. This cycle of three compounds was repeated a second time and thus was named *bi-cycle* or BIKE. Patients treated by either VAMP or BIKE had similar patterns of recurrence after therapy was discontinued, and both protocols produced unmaintained remissions significantly longer than those achieved when only prednisone was used for remission induction. Nevertheless, among 23 patients who completed the consolidation treatment, leukemia had recurred in 20 within 35 weeks of the end of therapy.[31,33]

By the early 1960s, the compounds known to be capable of inducing complete remission in children with ALL were prednisone, vincristine, 6-MP, methotrexate, and cyclophosphamide. Freireich and Frei stated that the effects on the leukemic process of these five remission-inducing agents are independent. Thus, the response or lack of response of a given patient's disease to any one agent does not affect the response to another. This might suggest that sequential use of available drugs would be optimal. They concluded, however, that "patients who fail to respond to a given agent have a probability of death from complications, so that the chance of surviving to receive the next compound diminishes progressively with each therapeutic regimen. This, as well as the possibility of drug synergism or potentiation, led to the study of these agents in combination."[13]

A major reason that all patients do not respond to therapy is that toxicity limits the amount of a drug that can be used. In combination therapy, a highly toxic agent can be combined with one of low toxicity. Prednisone and vincristine cause little or no marrow depression, so a combination of these two or of one of these with 6-MP, methotrexate, or cyclophosphamide should permit full dosage of each compound to be given simultaneously. The frequency of remission from a combination is always higher than that from any one agent; for example, the rate for the combination of prednisone (60 percent when given alone) and vincristine (55 percent alone) is 85 percent.[13]

POMP

Immediately after the VAMP and BIKE investigations, a third trial using combination chemotherapy was undertaken. Higher doses were administered for shorter periods, and the four remission-inducing agents were prednisone, vincristine [Oncovin], methotrexate, and 6-MP [Purinethol] (POMP).[31] As Henderson stated, "The current protocol is an intensification of the combination chemotherapy of the VAMP protocol and includes in addition to the early remission treatment intermittent monthly 'pulses' of combination drug therapy for the subsequent one year."[34]

Between 1962 and 1965, combination therapy with multiple agents was administered at the St. Jude Children's Research Hospital to 37 children who had ALL. After 5 years, 8 children were still living. In 7 of the 8, disease was in complete remission when the report was published; they had not received any therapy for 1½ to 3½ years. Pinkel's "total therapy" regime consisted of four phases:

1. induction of complete remission with prednisone and vincristine;
2. high doses of antimetabolite compounds injected intravenously every day for 1 week;
3. cerebrospinal irradiation; and
4. prolonged combination chemotherapy over 2 to 3 years.[35]

In 1967, both the systemic and the cerebrospinal therapies were intensified, with significant improvement in outcome. Of 35 children who had previously untreated ALL, 31 achieved complete remissions. Of these 31 patients, 18 were alive and free of leukemia in 1986, which was 18 years after diagnosis and 16 years after stopping all treatment.[36]

MOPP

As Zubrod remembered:

In 1963 DeVita, Moxley and Frei developed the first 4-drug combination for Hodgkin's disease.
The first combination MOMP (cyclophosphamide, vincristine, methotrexate and prednisone) was used together with irradiation. The first patient was treated September 27, 1963. In 1965, DeVita gave a paper on the results in the first 14 patients.[37] While MOMP was highly effective, procarbazine had recently been shown to have activity and it was substituted for methotrexate. The resulting MOPP combination

[Mustargen, Oncovin, procarbazine, prednisone] was given to the first patient at [the] NCI on August 5, 1964.[38]

Data on the first 43 patients, who had advanced Hodgkin's disease, demonstrated that MOPP had quadrupled the complete remission rate to 81 percent and had prolonged relapse-free survival.[39] The limiting toxicity was mainly bone marrow suppression.

In a 10-year progress report, DeVita et al. stated that, between 1964 and 1976, 194 patients with advanced Hodgkin's disease had been treated with the MOPP schedule. The complete remission rate was still 81 percent, and 66 percent of these persons had remained in remission at 5- and 10-year follow-ups. No patient had relapsed after 42 months off therapy, and no one who had failed induction therapy survived 5 years.[40]

The dramatic results of MOPP remained unsurpassed until the 1980s, when it became apparent that other drugs were effective against Hodgkin's disease; four of these (Adriamycin, bleomycin, vinblastine, dimethyltriazenoimidazole carboxamide [DTIC]) were combined in the ABVD regimen.[41] This combination was developed as an alternative for patients refractory to MOPP. When it was seen that results were equivalent to those of MOPP, two studies in which a course of MOPP was alternated with a course of ABVD were conducted.[42,43] In both of these trials, the complete remission rates (approaching 92 percent) were higher than those achieved with MOPP alone. This regimen has been used primarily for persons with advanced stages III and IV disease.

Ara-C Combination Therapy

Although the early trials of combination chemotherapy were conducted in children who had ALL, by the late 1960s, when the beneficial effects of Ara-C in AML had been documented, various combinations were also administered against that disorder. The same basic principles were followed even though the agents, the combinations, and the schedules differed.

The first combination therapy using Ara-C was reported by Gee et al. in 1969. They treated 40 adults suffering from myeloblastic leukemia with daily i.v. injections of Ara-C plus oral thioguanine. Among the 36 evaluable patients, the median survival was 11 months and that of the 19 responders was over 19 months.[44]

Describing a trial from St. Bartholomew's Hospital, London, Crowther et al. reported on the combination of cytosine arabinoside and daunorubicin for remission-induction chemotherapy of adults with AML (1970). An intensive intermittent regimen produced complete remissions in 14 of 23 patients (60 percent).[45] Physicians have been very successful with this combination over the years, and it continues to be a component of frontline therapy for AML.

During the 1970s and 1980s, the most commonly used regimens for remission induction in patients who had AML were combinations based on Ara-C (see chapter 4). Before about 1966, objective complete hematologic remissions were achieved in less than 10 percent of persons who had AML. The life span for the average patient was less than 4 months, and over 90 percent of patients died of their disease within a year of starting treatment. It was not unusual to have debates on the subject "should acute myelogenous leukemia be treated?"[46]

Combination chemotherapy was in use for ALL from about the mid-1960s, and it soon became apparent that prolonged survival was achieved only in the group attaining remissions. Among patients with AML who were treated at the NCI between 1955 and 1966, 50 percent of the persons who achieved remissions lived 10.5 months, compared with only 3.5 months for those who did not respond to remission-induction therapy. Median survival (of all patients), however, showed a minimal increase of 1 month (from 5 to 6 months). At Memorial Sloan-Kettering Cancer Center between 1951 and 1966, 25 percent of patients who had AML achieved complete or partial remissions with single agents, but there was no significant influence on the overall median survival of 4.5 months.[47-49]

It was in this atmosphere that Crosby in 1968 wrote his controversial editorial questioning the judgment of treating patients, who were doomed to an early death, with extremely toxic chemicals that might, themselves, be fatal.[50] In the zealous airing of pros and cons that followed,[51-54] it was generally acknowledged that, although treatment should not, if possible, harm patients, there was a need for specialized centers to conduct further research along protocol lines.[47]

Ara-C-based regimens for AML now result in complete remission rates of 50 to 90 percent and in cure rates of 15 to 40 percent, depending on population characteristics.[55-58] Although a high percentage of patients achieve complete remission, the paramount task is maintaining the remission. The relapse rate is particularly high during the first 18 months of remission. Although prolonged maintenance chemotherapy has been very successful in childhood ALL, the problem of short duration of remission in AML still exists.

MENINGEAL LEUKEMIA

After the introduction of the antimetabolites, patients, particularly children, who had ALL frequently experienced prolonged hematologic remissions, and many relapsed with meningeal leukemia.[59,60] This complication was occurring more frequently not only because these agents were prolonging the life span but also because they failed to reach therapeutic levels in the cerebrospinal fluid. The leukemic cells found a pharmacologic sanctuary in the central nervous system. The patient's peripheral blood could be completely normal during convulsions from meningeal leukemia.

Sansone (1954) was the first to report the use of intrathecal aminopterin. He treated two children suffering from meningeal leukemia and achieved moderate results.[61,62] He noted specifically that the neurologic symptoms occurred during a period of complete hematologic remission.

The clinical syndrome of meningeal leukemia was described precisely only after the advent of effective antileukemic therapy. Over the 70-year period from 1878 to 1948, 31 cases were reported. In contrast, during the 10-year interval after chemotherapy was introduced (1949 to 1959), descriptions of 69 cases were published.[63]

Sullivan (1957) reported that approximately one fourth of the children with leukemia followed at M. D. Anderson over an 18-month period had develped increased intracranial pressure, often with severe headache, vomiting, and papilledema. She wrote that therapy with "roentgen rays to the entire skull" was an effective treatment.[60]

Cranial irradiation and/or intrathecal methotrexate was used as therapy or prophylaxis against meningeal leukemia. Soon, however, investigators began reporting serious neurologic damage in patients receiving intrathecal methotrexate.[64] Kay and colleagues (1971) wrote that during or shortly after a course of intrathecal methotrexate therapy some patients developed "confusion, irritability, somnolence, ataxia, and dementia with major epileptic fits in two cases, and progression to coma and death in one."[65] When the condition was recognized, administration of folic and folinic acids arrested the progress of the syndrome, but they feared residual deficits such as partial blindness or intellectual impairment.[64,65]

In 1960, physicians at the NCI reported 25 cases of meningeal leukemia among 150 consecutively admitted patients with acute leukemia. After diffuse leukemic cells infiltrate the arachnoid,[66] fluid pressure increases and symmetrical hydrocephalus involves all four ventricles. The cranial sutures spread in children, and they may develop papilledema, vomiting, headaches, convulsions, or cranial nerve palsies. Neurologists at the NCI would not allow lumbar puncture because of the danger of herniation. However, because these children were dying and the attending physicians were desperate to help, it was decided to try a puncture; a neurosurgeon stood by in case burr holes in the skull became necessary. The spinal fluid was under increased pressure and there was pleocytosis of leukemic cells, but no herniation occurred because the communicating hydrocephalus equalized pressure throughout the system. Thereafter, all patients with signs and symptoms of meningeal leukemia had spinal taps (sometimes several).

The article written by these physicians was rejected by three journals and finally appeared in *Neurology*.[63] It was important because it described a definite clinical syndrome that could be diagnosed in life. Rieselbach and associates (1962) used intrathecal aminopterin plus citrovorum factor protection to treat 15 patients who had ALL and had experienced 24 episodes of meningeal leukemia. All patients achieved remissions of meningeal leukemia, but even more significant was the fact that systemic leukemia was markedly improved.[62] This observation stimulated the parenteral use of methotrexate.

Subsequently, long-term, possibly irreversible, adverse effects from cranial irradiation were reported, and the prospect of such complications led to trials of many variations in therapy; numerous different doses and schedules have been tested. Studies over the years have clearly revealed that all children with ALL, even those considered to be at low risk for central nervous system relapse, should receive some prophylactic therapy. Bleyer (1988) summarized: "On a worldwide basis, chemoradiotherapy with cranial radiotherapy and intrathecal methotrexate remains the established method of preventing overt central nervous system leukemia. The benefits of this intervention, in terms of prevention of symptomatic central nervous system leukemia, prolongation of complete remission, and increased cure rates, are clearly worth the risks."[67]

SIX

Supportive Therapy

'Tis not enough to help the feeble up,
but to support him after.

WILLIAM SHAKESPEARE (1564–1616), *Timon of Athens,*
act 1, scene 1, line 108

When treating patients with leukemia, success or failure in achieving remission frequently depends on the supportive care provided during the symptomatic periods. Hemorrhage and infection are major threats to survival, and it is imperative that physicians anticipate and forestall these possibilities or institute appropriate treatment promptly. Blood transfusions and radiation were about the only therapies available for leukemia until the late 1940s. Today, however, in addition to chemotherapy, an array of supportive measures are available, including platelet or leukocyte replacement, antibiotics, protected environments, biologic response modifiers, and bone marrow transplantation.

TRANSFUSIONS

Whole Blood Transfusion

From primitive times, blood was regarded as the most fundamental element of life itself; a person's blood was supposed to carry the hidden components of his or her basic personality, the person's individuality. Thus, it is not surprising that many references to blood appear in the Bible. Some of these have been interpreted by Jehovah's Witnesses as God's forbidding blood transfusion. For example, "Whatsoever man there be of the house of Israel, or of the strangers that sojourn among you, that catch any manner of blood: I will even set my face against that soul that eateth blood, and will cut him off from among his people" (Lev. 17:10).

In the Middle Ages, blood was often ingested to strengthen the body. Some writers have stated that the first blood transfusion was administered in 1492 to Pope Innocent VIII after a stroke. The blood was supposedly obtained by bleeding three boys to death. Because it was not known at that time that blood circulates, it seems more likely that the blood must have been administered as a draught.[1] However, the publication of the theory of the circulation of the blood by William Harvey in 1628 led inevitably to the invention of methods to transfer blood from a vigorous to a debilitated subject.

The first successful blood transfusions on lower animals were performed by Richard Lower in 1665.[1,2] Lower was a pioneer experimental physiologist known for making one of the greatest discoveries in the history of medicine, recognizing that blood changes color by deriving some "quality" when passing through the lungs. Lower connected an artery of one animal to a vein of another by means of a pipe.[1] In 1981, Oberman wrote:[3]

> It seems clear that Lower was the first to define the appropriateness of transfusional replacement of blood in severe hemorrhage, since he was able to demonstrate that a dog could be exsanguinated to the point of death and then be completely restored by transfusion. It is interesting to note that a contemporary record of this experiment is contained in the diary of Samuel Pepys. His entry of November 14, 1666 notes: "Dr. Croone told me that, at the meeting at Gresham College tonight there was a pretty experiment of the blood of one dog let out till he died, into the body of another on one side, while all his own run out on the other side. The first died upon the place, and the other very well and likely to do well. This did give occasion to many pretty wishes, as of the blood of a Quaker

to be let into an Archbishop, and such like; but, as Dr. Croone says, may, if it takes, be of mighty use to a man's health, for the amendment of bad blood by borrowing from a better body."[4]

At that time, blood was still regarded as the carrier of an animal's characteristics. This was evidenced by the fact that, in 1666, Robert Boyle wrote to Dr. Lower to speculate about the possible effect of cross-transfusion: "as whether the blood of a mastiff, being frequently transfused into a bloodhound, or a spaniel, will not prejudice them in point of scent."[5]

Jean Baptiste Denis (or Denys),[6] a young physician to King Louis XIV, read of Lower's work in the *Journal des Savants* of January 31, 1667. He initiated his own trials with dogs. According to Brown (1948):

> On June 13, [1667], the Journal reviewed a pamphlet by Claude Tardy,[7] who sees various possibilities in the procedure, especially on man, and suggests transfusion from vein to vein, and the limiting of the quantity of blood to be taken from the donor. From this the old may be rejuvenated, and cures obtained in diseases arising from the "acrimonius state of the blood," such as ulcers and erysipelas, on which ordinary medicines work slowly because their strength is lost before they reach the blood stream. A fresh, well-tempered blood going directly into the affected parts, he thinks, should work much more effectively than anything else yet suggested; nor is it necessary to rely on human blood, as that of a calf or other animal is likely to produce a similar effect.[8]

This may be the first published text presenting a function for human transfusion. No previous writings had suggested a logical or beneficial outcome.

On June 15, 1667, the first blood transfusion to a human was documented:[8]

> The first patient, a boy of 15 or 16, had suffered for two months with a stubborn fever, for which he had been bled some twenty times; now heavy and lethargic, he had lost his memory, and become quite stupid. He fell asleep at meals, which seemed to show that the small amount of blood remaining in his veins had been thickened by the fever; in general, Denis thought a

transfusion might be advantageous. The surgeon, Emerez, drew off about three ounces from a vein at the elbow, the blood being dark and thick; and the patient received about eight ounces of arterial blood from a lamb's carotid. The boy immediately felt relieved from the pain of a bruise suffered on the day before falling from a ladder; his lethargy passed, he became gay and cheerful as he had been before his illness, ate well, and slept in more reasonable proportions.[9]

The boy continued to make a remarkable recovery. Denis transfused blood into several other persons that same year and frequently noted that, after the procedure, the patient passed urine as black as soot. This was, of course, due to hemoglobinuria, resulting from massive hemagglutination and hemolysis.[1]

A 34-year-old mental patient, Antoine Mauroy, had a hemolytic reaction after his second transfusion. Denis' description is rated as a medical classic:[10]

As soon as the blood began to enter into his veins, he felt the heat along his arm and under his armpits. His pulse rose and soon after we observed a plentiful sweat over all his face. His pulse varied extremely at this instant and he complained of great pains in his kidneys, and that he was ready to choke unless given his liberty. He was made to lie down and fell asleep, and slept all night without awakening until morning. When he awakened he made a great glass full of urine, of a color as black as if it had been mixed with the soot of chimneys.[3]

M. Mauroy died during his third transfusion and a lengthy court case ensued. Denis was finally exonerated, but, eventually, blood transfusion was forbidden in France and the procedure was set aside.

During the following 168 years there seems to have been little interest in blood transfusion. The chief obstacle had always been coagulation of the blood.[1] In 1835, however, Bischoff overcame this problem by using defibrinated blood.[1,11] This advance led to the invention of many ingenious instruments for transfusion. The apparatus used by Sir Thomas Smith (as published in *Lancet*, 1873) consisted of the following paraphernalia: "a wire egg-beater, a hair sieve, a three-ounce glass aspirator syringe, a fine blunt-ended aspirator canula with a lateral and a terminal opening, a short piece of india-rubber tubing with a brass nozzle at either end connecting the syringe with the canula, a tall narrow vessel standing in warm water for defibrinating the blood, and a suitable vessel floated in warm water to contain the defibrinated blood."[12]

Severe symptoms and fatalities, which must have been the results of using blood from incompatible donors, continued to occur. Before 1900, physicians knew that a transfusion could cause a fatal reaction in a recipient, but they could offer no explanation for such a response. In that year, Landsteiner,[1,13] and independently Shattock,[1,14] reported the presence of isoagglutinins in the blood. When the red blood cells from one individual are mixed with the serum from a person of an incompatible blood type, massive clumping of the cells results, an occurrence termed *isoagglutination*.

Janský (1907) showed that human blood can be classified into four groups on the basis of the agglutinins and agglutinable substances it contains.[1,15] Crile (1907) described a feasible procedure for transfusing blood directly.[16] He drew the vein of the recipient through a small cannula and cuffed it back over the tube. The donor's artery was eased over the vein, and thus there was an uninterrupted intima coat, leaving no rough surfaces to cause coagulation.[1] Crile reported an extensive series of experimental transfusions in dogs in his monograph, *Hemorrhage and Transfusion* (1909).[17] His innovative work heralded the use of transfusion as a practical therapeutic measure, and Crile deserves the credit for the subsequent popularity of the process.[1]

Von Ziemssen had, in 1892, accomplished blood transfer by rapidly drawing 20 ml of blood from the donor's vein, disconnecting the syringe from the needle, and emptying it through a needle (previously inserted in the recipient's vein) before coagulation intervened. By filling the syringes, one after another, he could transfuse as much as 280 ml at one time.[1,18] Lindeman (1913) altered this method by using many syringes, kept constantly washed by an assistant, and sets of three cannulas that telescoped one within the other. In expert hands, the method yielded good results, but it was unwieldy and required practice for the team of workers to become adept.[1,19] This contribution is of historic importance because it led to the invention of an improved syringe with a two-way stopcock (Unger, 1915).[20]

Defibrination of blood was not simple or satisfactory, and a major advance was made by Hustin of Belgium (1914) when he used a glucose and sodium citrate solution as an anticoagulant.[1,21] Agote performed the first transfusion in which citrated blood alone was used on November 14, 1914, in Buenos Aires.[1,22]

As soon as blood transfusion became practicable, it was, and it still is, used to replace blood loss or to improve levels of all blood elements in patients who have leukemia. To our knowledge, keeping the hemoglobin as close as possible to a normal value does not aid in white blood cell recovery in neutropenic patients.

Although the possibility of AIDS infection via transfusion exists, at present it does not seem to be a major problem for patients who have leukemia. They usually receive blood donations from family members, and all donated blood is screened meticulously.

Platelet Transfusion

Duke (1910), in a landmark article, was the first to delineate the importance of platelets in hemorrhagic disease. He reported

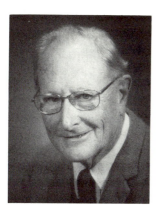

that the platelet count was elevated and bleeding was temporarily stopped after direct transfusion to thrombopenic patients. In the same paper, Duke described the original bleeding-time test that bears his name and is still in use today.[23]

According to Cohn, the Italian school, early in the twentieth century, recommended blood transfusion for thrombocytopenic purpura.[24] Because suitable anticoagulants were not available, paraffin-coated syringes were used.[25] Occasional accounts of plate-

Eugene P. Cronkite

let transfusions were published before 1950, but most patients with thrombocytopenia received fresh whole blood, preferably from donors with thrombocytosis.

The incidence of thrombocytopenic purpura was high at Hiroshima and Nagasaki after the atomic bombings, and it was realized that this could be a significant complication of modern warfare.[25] A low platelet count is the principal cause of bleeding after whole-body exposure to penetrating, ionizing radiation.[26] The atomic bomb provided the impetus for some of the research and development of platelet preservation and use. Cronkite and colleagues performed extensive studies on the separation and transfusion of platelets to treat radiation hemorrhage in animals.[25-31]

Hirsch et al. (1950) reported a case of chronic idiopathic thrombocytopenia in which the patient's platelets were not only reduced in number but also morphologically abnormal and physiologically defective. Transfusion of blood from a polycythemic donor whose platelet count was about eight times the normal level resulted in the recovery of a detectable proportion of these platelets in the patient. The donor platelets survived 5 to 6 days and retained their normal physiologic activity.[32]

Hirsch and Gardner (1952) studied platelet recovery in recipients, the life span of transfused platelets, and the clinical effect of transfusing platelets. They described 42 transfusions of polycythemic or normal blood without anticoagulants to 35 thrombocytopenic persons by means of multiple silicone-coated syringes. These transfusions effectively raised the platelet counts temporarily and caused spontaneous bleeding to cease. The transfused platelets remained in the circulation of patients with bone marrow aplasia for 5 to 6 days.[33]

Brecher et al. (1953), using venous blood collected in siliconed test tubes, showed that platelet counts made under a phase microscope were reproducible and relatively accurate.[34] This method was later used by Gaydos and colleagues (1962) to demonstrate a quantitative relationship between the frequency of hemorrhage and the platelet count. In a study using capillary blood from 92 persons with acute leukemia, they found that hemorrhage was more prevalent and more severe among those with lower platelet levels. No "threshold level" was apparent, but gross bleeding occurred rarely when counts were above 20,000 per cu mm.[35]

By the late 1950s, however, in spite of the development of plastic and other nonwettable surfaces and the capability of transfusing viable platelets, such transfusions were not used as standard therapeutic procedure. This was primarily because of the difficulty in finding large numbers of available donors and because of the lengthy manipulations necessary for preparing platelet concentrates. Freireich and associates (1959) reported that fresh blood was more effective than banked blood in alleviating hemorrhage in persons with acute leukemia. Patients' platelet levels were significantly higher after fresh-blood transfusions.[36]

Zubrod later recalled that, during this period, platelet transfusions were not generally accepted.

> Hematologists had shown, using labeled (and therefore damaged) platelets, that infused platelets did not last more than a few hours. Freireich and Frei showed that most of the fatal hemorrhages occurred when the platelet count fell to <20,000/cu mm and that fresh whole blood (containing undamaged platelets) could raise the count to >20,000 and prevent fatal hemorrhage. Then there was a series of studies to harvest and preserve platelets. These studies were vigorously attacked by classical hematologists because they required larger amounts of blood than blood banks could easily obtain. I recall a dramatic showdown at a clinical staff meeting in 1956 where a motion was made to deny platelets to the NCI. . . . The other clinical directors came to our support and the motion was narrowly defeated. . . . Later the NCI studies unequivocally demonstrated the great value of platelets in preventing hemorrhage and platelet transfusion became one of the major elements in keeping patients with leukemia alive until complete remission could be induced.[37]

In time, physicians came to realize that thrombocytopenia was of primary importance in patients who were bleeding.

By 1963, plasmapheresis had been shown to increase the quantity of platelet-rich plasma produced by each donor by at least 50-fold; the yield of a single donor could reach 2 liters per week.[38] Freireich and colleagues wrote that platelet survival depends to a major degree on the clinical status of the recipient; the presence of fever and infection, especially, results in poor platelet survival. They found that transfusions of platelet-rich plasma stopped hemorrhage in 51 of 57 instances. The duration of hemostasis was related to the length of time that the posttransfusion platelet count remained elevated.[38]

Djerassi and colleagues also reported in 1963 that platelet concentrates stopped bleeding in 20 of 33 patients. A consistent and significant elevation of circulating platelets occurred when 0.08 unit or more of platelets per pound of body weight was transfused. However, the increased platelet count rarely persisted for more than 24 hours.[39] Alvarado et al. (1965) wrote that fresh concentrated platelets controlled overt bleeding on 15 of 25 occasions in children with acute leukemia. With the exception of melena, all bleeding was arrested when the platelet count was increased by more than 40,000 platelets/cu mm. Survival of platelets was short in patients with active disease and in those with infection.[40]

Menitove, in 1983, described a problem: "Most haematologists and oncologists prescribe platelet transfusions prophylactically to prevent bleeding for their patients with platelet counts below 20,000/cu mm. One risk that accompanies this policy is the development of alloimmunization. This has been estimated to occur in 70–100 percent of patients."[41]

Many investigators recognized this problem—that a significant proportion of persons who received multiple platelet transfusions developed antibodies against antigens on the platelets, and these antibodies rapidly destroyed the transfused platelets. This is called the *refractory state*. It is now known that approximately two thirds of the patients who receive random-donor platelets develop alloantibodies and do not respond to the platelet transfusions.[42] Refractoriness associated with alloimmunity can be reversed, however, by using platelets obtained from donors whose human leukocyte antigen (HLA) type matches that of the recipient.[41]

It is possible to collect platelets from patients with acute leukemia while they are in remission and freeze and store the platelets for subsequent use. The process is expensive, and the posttransfusion recovery rate is lower than that after transfusion of fresh platelets. However, some centers use this method and find it helpful for patients who become alloimmunized during induction therapy.[41]

McCredie et al. (1974) stated:

The development of . . . plateletpheresis, in which platelet-poor plasma is returned to the donor, has made it possible to collect multiple units of platelets from individual donors, who can donate platelets repeatedly at short intervals without risk. . . .

The most difficult problem has been preserving the platelet. . . .

The process of concentrating platelets from platelet-rich plasma can cause them to aggregate, . . . [producing decreased] viability.[43]

Discovering the details of the platelet aggregation reaction led to the demonstration that acidifying the plasma before concentrating it protected against clumping.[44]

Storage of platelets was another problem to be solved. In 1985, Murphy explained that, "in the years preceding 1970, platelets for transfusion were stored under refrigeration at 4°C. After only 8 hours of such storage, survival after infusion was measurably compromised, and after 18 hours, mean platelet survival was markedly reduced, to 1–2 days (the value for fresh platelets is 6–10 days). Thus, storage beyond 24 hours was unacceptable.[45] In the early 1970s, however, it was recognized that, if platelets were stored for 1 week at room temperature (20–24°C), mean platelet survival time was only trivially reduced. In the beginning, storage was of platelet-rich plasma, but soon platelet concentrates were made and stored. Containers were of polyvinylchloride plastic, and after 3 days of storage, the platelet concentrates often had a pH below 6. In 1975, it was reported that the pH remained higher when storage was in polyolefin containers.[46] At present, modifications of these containers offer blood banks the means to store platelet concentrates for 1 week with acceptable viability and function.[45]

The major risk of platelet transfusion is hepatitis transmission. Posttransfusion hepatitis will develop in 2 to 10 percent of blood recipients.[47] However, in patients exposed to multiple donors and who receive both pooled platelets and red blood cells, the risk is considerably higher, probably exceeding 40 percent.[47–49]

Leukocyte Replacement

With the development of feasible separation techniques for blood components, physicians were able by the early 1970s to select the constituent required. Because hemorrhage could be prevented and treated with platelet transfusions, infection became the major cause of death in patients with acute leukemia. Correlation is strong between the degree and duration of granulocytopenia and the susceptibility to severe infection. Also, effective replacement of white blood cells should lead to more effective chemotherapy because the limiting factor in chemotherapy and extended-field radiotherapy is severe bone marrow depression.[50]

The earliest reference we could find to human leukocyte replacement therapy was that of Strumia from 1934. He described his method for making "leucocyte cream":

> normally stimulation to new granulocytic cell formation is due to material liberated from the breaking down of old cells. Very likely the beneficial effect of transfusions in neutropenias is due to the introduction in circulation of such material.
>
> . . . leucocytic cream intramuscularly in severe neutropenias is followed in most cases within one to four days, usually 48 hours, by an increase in mature granulocytic cells in circulation, along with a considerable clinical improvement.[51]

The main obstacles to white blood cell transfusion are (1) the low yield of leukocytes when blood is centrifuged and (2) the short half-life of granulocytes. We can measure the half-life of transfused red blood cells in weeks (or months) and that of transfused platelets in days. The half-life of a circulating granulocyte is 4 to 6 hours.[50] Patients with CML who had granulocyte counts 30 to 50 times normal have been used as donors by plasmapheresis. These transfusions to patients with granulocytopenia have resulted in reduction of fever, cure of septicemia, healing of acute and chronic lesions, and eradication of bacterial infection.[50] A 1975 report of the original studies using donors with CML cited an approximately 70 percent neutropenia cure rate.[52]

On rare occasions, recipients of transfusions from donors with CML have developed chronic myelogenous leukemic cell allografts. Also, because of the restricted number of donors with CML and because repeated plasmapheresis failed to reduce their white blood cell counts significantly, it was necessary to investigate other possibilities for obtaining granulocytes.[50] A continuous-flow blood-cell separator was invented to facilitate processing large volumes of blood from normal donors as well as from those who had CLL or CML.

In 1970, histocompatibility testing for leukocyte transfusions was reported.[53] When donor and recipient were matched for HLA type, the median transfused-leukocyte recovery at 1 hour post-transfusion was 24 percent; with mismatches the 1-hour recovery is approximately 5 percent.[50]

Prophylactic leukocyte transfusions have been used for patients who have newly diagnosed leukemia and also for bone marrow transplant recipients. Winston and colleagues (UCLA) found that these persons had significantly more cytomegalovirus infections after transfusion than did control patients receiving no leukocytes or only therapeutic leukocyte transfusions. The authors believed that these findings were consistent with the hypothesis that latent cytomegalovirus may be present in leukocytes of blood donors with previous cytomegalovirus infection and after transfusion may be activated to produce an active infection.[54]

Bodey stated that in recent years the availability of more effective antibiotic regimens has reduced the need for granulocyte transfusions. They are still used, although their efficacy remains controversial.[54] Seventy-five to 85 percent of infected neutropenic patients will improve with prompt administration of broad spectrum antibiotics alone,[55,56] and Bodey recommends that granulocyte transfusions should be used only for those patients who fail to respond to appropriate antibiotics.[57]

ANTIBIOTICS

Antibacterial Agents

Chemotherapy for leukemia has extended life and even accomplished cures in many instances. Most patients, however, experience side effects from the drugs, and these reactions may themselves be extremely grave and even fatal. Most of the agents used against leukemia cause varying degrees of myelosuppression that may lead to an extreme and extended neutropenia. As a result, treated patients are very vulnerable to infections from an assortment of virulent organisms, and infection continues to be a paramount complication. It is not rare for someone to succumb to infection before an effective dosage of chemotherapy can be administered. In addition, physicians are often forced to reduce the dosage or length of time the patient receives chemotherapeutic agents because infection ensues. However, effective antibiotic therapy has frequently made it possible to administer the more aggressive chemotherapeutic regimens that have cured some cancers.

In the mid-1950s, physicians at the NCI concentrated efforts on promptly identifying pathogens responsible for infections and treating them with massive antibiotic combinations. Zubrod subsequently wrote that these measures paid off in terms of fewer deaths from infections.[37] The fundamental and innovative approach developed at the Institute at that time was summarized by Bodey: "Antibiotic therapy should be administered to the neutropenic patient promptly at the onset of fever, after the culture specimens have been obtained. If therapy is delayed until the infecting organism has been identified, a substantially greater portion of these infections will be fatal."[58] Antibiotics against the major organisms that cause death were prescribed empirically.

Two early prospective randomized trials of adjunct therapy to supplement antibiotics for patients with acute leukemia were conducted by Bodey et al. at the NCI. In 1964, 46 of these patients who were having episodes of fever were randomly allocated to receive either antibiotics and gamma globulin (treatment group) or antibiotics alone (control group). The antibiotics used were sodium methicillin and sodium colistimethate (Coly-Mycin). No significant benefit was derived from the use of gamma globulin.[59]

In a second trial, the effects of corticosteroids and gamma globulin, in addition to antibiotics, were studied in patients who had infections complicating acute leukemia. Patients were randomly assigned to receive antibiotics alone (group 1), antibiotics and gamma globulin (group 2), or antibiotics plus gamma globulin and steroids (group 3). Patients in group 3 had a slightly higher cure rate, a somewhat lower death rate and incidence of shock, and a shorter duration of illness.[60] The vast majority of organisms cultured were either gram-negative bacilli or fungi.

Also, it soon became apparent that, although some antibiotics (colistin and polymyxin B) were very active in vitro against gram-negative bacilli, they were ineffective in neutropenic patients. In trials, aminoglycosides were substituted, but the investigators quickly learned that these, as well, had only a weak influence in neutropenic persons.

For example, in a retrospective study of *Pseudomonas* bacteremia in patients with severe neutropenia (<100/cu mm), the cure rate was 70 percent if patients received a beta lactam antibiotic (frequently carbenicillin) as a single agent, but only 17 percent if they received an aminoglycoside as the only antipseudomonal drug.[61]

This same study revealed the importance of prescribing the proper antibiotic at the onset of the infection. When patients did not receive appropriate antibiotic therapy at the outset, 15 percent died within 12 hours of drawing blood for the first positive culture, 57 percent within 24 hours, and over 70 percent within 48 hours. Among patients who received antipseudomonal therapy, the cure rate was 74 percent when the therapy was given promptly at the time the blood for culture was drawn; when treatment was delayed 1 to 2 days, the cure rate was only 46 percent.[57,61]

Carbenicillin was the first antipseudomonal penicillin; before its introduction, the only agents available for treating *Pseudomonas* infections were polymyxins and, later, gentamicin. These were not effective in combating *Pseudomonas* infections in neutropenic patients, who sustained a fatality rate in excess of 75 percent. Occasionally, the infection subsided in persons whose neutrophil counts improved as their leukemia went into remission. In the early 1970s, patients fared no better with antibiotic therapy than without it. Fewer than 20 percent of patients with *Pseudomonas* septicemia responded to polymyxin B, and the mortality was approximately 90 percent.[62]

Bodey and colleagues (1969, 1971) conducted the first trials of carbenicillin in neutropenic patients and demonstrated an extraordinary improvement. The drug was effective in 91 percent of infectious episodes caused by *Pseudomonas*, even in patients with severe neutropenia. However, 7 percent of patients had only partial improvement and 10 percent relapsed when therapy was discontinued. The response rate for *E. coli* infections was 58 percent.[63,64]

After gentamicin was introduced, carbenicillin alone and gentamicin alone were compared with a combination of the two by Klastersky and associates (1973). Their trial cohort consisted of patients with disseminated cancer and life-threatening infections. Patients were randomized into one of the three treatment groups, and the antibiotic was started at the time of a presumed diagnosis of sepsis by gram-negative rods. Favorable results were achieved in 50 percent of those receiving carbenicillin alone, in 57 percent of those receiving gentamicin alone, and in 83 percent of those receiving the combination.[65] This lower response rate for carbenicillin alone, when compared with the previous study, may

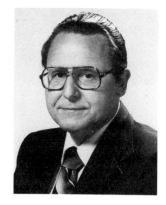

Gerald P. Bodey

have been the result of the schedule of administration, which was suboptimal considering the drug's half-life.[62]

When ticarcillin was developed, Rodriguez et al. (1973) reported that 16 of 20 episodes caused by *Pseudomonas* were cured, as were 3 of 3 infections due to *Proteus* species and 1 resulting from *Haemophilus influenzae*.[66] However, the drug performed poorly when infections were caused by *E. coli*, *Klebsiella* species, *Enterobacter* species, *Salmonella* species, and mixed organisms, indicating a limited range of action. Eventually, combination therapy with carbenicillin or ticarcillin plus an aminoglycoside or cephalothin became the accepted regime.[62]

In 1965, Hersh et al. reported the leading causes of death of 414 patients with acute leukemia treated at the NCI. These persons died during the 10-year period from 1954 to 1963. The number of fatal hemorrhages declined markedly over this time span, as did the number of fatal staphylococcal infections. At the same time, fatal infections caused by fungi increased dramatically.[67] The decline in staphylococcal infections was related to the introduction of methicillin, the first antistaphylococcal semisynthetic penicillin. (In recent years, a *S. aureus* that is resistant to methicillin has appeared at some institutions.[68])

Both incidence and severity of infection are inversely related to the level of circulating neutrophils in patients with acute leukemia. Virtually every patient who spends more than 3 weeks with a neutrophil level of <100/cu mm of blood contracts infection, and it disseminates widely and rapidly.[58]

Before the 1980s, the majority of infections in patients with neutropenia were caused by gram-negative bacilli (*Pseudomonas aeruginosa, E. coli, Klebsiella* species). In a 1978 study of 494 patients with acute leukemia, the pathogens were identified as aerobic gram-negative bacilli in 70 percent of 848 episodes of infection.[69] However, Pizzo and associates (1978) reported the increasing incidence of gram-positive sepsis in cancer patients,[70] and, during the 1980s, the resurgence of gram-positive infections has continued. The liberal use of indwelling catheters has contributed to this trend and has also been conducive to the appearance of new pathogens. In many institutions, infections in neutropenic patients are now caused chiefly by gram-positive organisms.[68]

The fatality rate for most severe infections complicating acute leukemia is related to the patient's inability to respond with an increased production of neutrophils.[71] In 1966, the fatality rate was reported as about 60 percent for patients with an initial neutrophil count of $<1,000$/cu mm of blood that failed to increase during the first week of a severe infection. In contrast, patients with a similar count who responded to their infection with an increased number of circulating neutrophils had a fatality rate of about 32 percent.[58] Although the prognosis for these patients was much better in the 1980s as a result of the availability of more effective antibiotics, the basic principle still applies.

In animal experiments, both antitumor agents and adrenal corticosteroids enhance susceptibility to bacterial, fungal, viral, and protozoal infections. Clinical studies suggest that these drugs affect humans similarly. Multiple-organism septicemia is especially frequent in patients with hematologic malignancies.[72] Because patients with low neutrophil counts are susceptible to infection caused by a wide variety of pathogens, broad-spectrum coverage with antibiotics is imperative to keep these persons alive.[57]

Antifungal Agents

Fungal infections have been increasing in frequency and account for about 25 percent of fatal infections in persons with acute leukemia. Before the 1960s, articles on fungal infections in patients with depressed immunity were sparse. In 1953, Craig and Farber cited 13 cases of disseminated visceral infection by various fungi among 175 cases of childhood acute leukemia autopsied since the inception of active antileukemia treatment. There were no cases in children with untreated leukemia.[73]

In 1962, Baker reviewed 261 autopsies performed after death from leukemia between 1930 and 1961. A total of 39 persons (15 percent) had complicating fungus infections, 11 severe enough to be regarded as the cause of death. Baker associated fungus infections with neutropenia. No fatal cases occurred between 1930 and 1953; all 11 occurred after 1953, suggesting that "some factor of modern therapy is responsible for the fatalities."[74]

Persons with acute leukemia are particularly susceptible to mycosis. In the past these infections appeared during the terminal stages of the disease, but recently they have been reported earlier.[75] Estey et al. (1982) reviewed the years 1973 to 1979 and found that, among patients receiving initial remission-induction therapy for AML, fungi, either alone or together with bacteria, were responsible for 37 percent of all fatal infections.[76]

Bodey stated that the most frequent fungal infection in cancer patients is disseminated candidiasis, which often presents as fever of unknown origin. Although systemic antifungal agents are available, it is very difficult to establish the diagnosis early and, as a result, only 15 to 30 percent of patients with disseminated candidiasis ever receive antifungal therapy.[57]

Louria et al. (1962) outlined the variations in clinical presentation of disseminated candidiasis: (1) a sudden onset of fever, chills, and tachycardia that can easily be mistaken for a bacterial infection; (2) a gradual onset of fever with no other specific symptoms; and (3) a steady, general physical decline that may not be distinguishable from deterioration resulting from the malignancy.[57,77] Also, the group at M. D. Anderson Cancer Center found that, among 188 patients who had systemic candidiasis, *Candida* species were cultured from blood specimens collected during the first 48 hours of infection from only 8 percent of the patients and during the first week from only 18 percent.[78]

This same group found that the principal factor affecting recovery from systemic candidiasis is improvement in the neutrophil count. There were no survivors among 93 patients with candidiasis and persistent neutropenia, even though some (25) received antifungal therapy. Among 24 persons who had neutropenia at the onset of infection but who recovered from it, 5 of 13 who received antifungal drugs were cured of the candidiasis. None of 11 persons who received no antifungal therapy survived.[78]

Catheter-related candidemia in immunocompromised patients is associated with a high incidence of disseminated candidiasis and a high mortality. Therefore, all immunocompromised patients should receive antifungal therapy, and their catheters should probably be removed.[75]

Highly effective therapy for systemic mycoses in neutropenic patients is currently not available.[75,79] Amphotericin B remains the best option, but its success rate leaves much to be desired and side effects, both short- and long-term, can be severe. Miconazole, ketoconazole, and 5-fluorocytosine are also used against candidiasis, but the predominant factor in achieving a cure in a patient with leukemia is attaining a remission of the leukemia.[75] A lipid-encapsulated (liposomal) amphotericin B is a new form that has demonstrated effectiveness against both candidiasis and aspergillosis. The initial trial, admittedly very small, was encouraging, and side effects were minor.[80]

Whereas *Candida* infections originate primarily in the gastrointestinal tract (or in the bloodstream directly via catheters), aspergillosis is an airborne infestation and the majority of cases have pulmonary or sinus involvement. Again, neutropenia is a major factor contributing to the infection, as is prolonged use of adrenal corticosteroids. Pulmonary disease may include pneumonia of various types, abscesses, cavities, emboli, or thrombosis. Hemoptysis may be a complication of some of these disorders. The less common sinus infections may invade soft tissue, cartilage, and bone, even progressing, occasionally, to involve the orbits and the brain.[75]

As in candidiasis, an early definite diagnosis is usually not possible. Nevertheless, the presenting findings can suggest aspergillosis, and diagnostic tests and therapy can be instituted promptly. Amphotericin B is the only antifungal drug with proven effectiveness against *Aspergillus*.[75] As this is an airborne infection, purification of the air (see "A Protected Environment," following section) is paramount in prophylaxis, especially in conjunction with intensive therapy regimens such as bone marrow transplantation.

Because the treatment of fungus infections is frequently unsatisfactory and disappointing, prophylactic measures against these pathogens are of utmost importance for neutropenic patients. Meunier included basic principles such as careful handwashing by patients and all attendants; optimal dental care; a restricted diet of cooked food because yeasts, rusts, and molds may exist on raw fruits and vegetables; and avoidance of vascular or urinary indwelling catheters as much as possible.[79] In addition, prophylaxis against *Candida* with various regimens of amphotericin B, nystatin, ketoconazole, and miconazole have been studied. The latter drug was poorly absorbed after oral administration and is now available for injection only. Results with the other three compounds have varied widely. Differences in study designs and drug dosages have made comparisons difficult, and very few controlled, randomized trials have been conducted. Meunier and Klastersky reported good results with intranasally administered amphotericin B for prophylaxis of aspergillosis.[81]

In recent years, the increased use of bone marrow transplantation has generated additional challenges for those who treat infectious diseases, particularly in the area of control of fungi and viruses such as cytomegalovirus and Epstein-Barr virus.[82-84] The eradication therapy given before transplantation has prolonged, injurious effects on cellular immunity.[57] During the immediate posttransplantation period, patients are neutropenic and at risk of infections caused by gram-negative bacilli and fungi. After engraftment, there are "deficiencies in cellular immunity due to graft-versus-host disease and immunosuppressive therapy. Late infectious complications include those caused by gram-positive cocci and DNA viruses (cytomegalovirus, herpes simplex, and varicella-zoster), as well as *Pneumocystis* pneumonia and nonspecific interstitial pneumonitis."[57]

Since the discovery of penicillin, more than 80 antibiotics have been developed. As mentioned previously, the usual procedure for neutropenic persons has been to prescribe various combinations of agents for broad coverage. The recent development of drugs with a wider range, however, has again made single-agent antibiotic therapy feasible.[62] Clinical trials of monotherapy as initial empiric treatment for febrile neutropenic cancer patients have been instituted, and some of the investigators have documented good results, especially against gram-negative infections. How-

ever, gram-positive organisms are again prevalent in these patients, and another antibiotic such as nafcillin or vancomycin
may be required to provide better coverage.[62] Further studies comparing these newer antibiotics with the customary approach using
two synergistic agents are necessary.

Thus, although various therapeutic options are available today,
the salient point is the urgent need for the antibiotic regimen to
include a beta-lactam antibiotic that is active against the infecting
organism; one cannot rely on an aminoglycoside alone because
these drugs are not very effective in neutropenic patients.

Today, between 80 and 90 percent of bacterial infections are
being cured, including about 40 to 60 percent in patients with
neutrophil counts persistently below 100. The major problem is
the fungal superinfections that occur in the patients with persistent neutropenia. During the course of the disease, the average
patient with leukemia has about 10 potentially fatal infections
before finally dying (frequently of a fatal infection).

A PROTECTED ENVIRONMENT

In 1956, Reyniers et al. observed that the average survival time
of germ-free rats was approximately twice that of conventional
rats after receiving total-body x-irradiation above 4 Gy (400 rad).[85]
In 1963, two other publications citing experiments with germ-
free mice appeared. Wilson confirmed the work of Reyniers, finding that germ-free mice survived 4 days longer than normal mice
after whole-body x-irradiation in the 5- to 10-Gy (hematopoietic
death) range.[86] White and Claflin reported that germ-free mice are
also more resistant to the delayed lethal consequences of nitrogen
mustard than are regular mice.[87]

These experiments showed that germ-free animals could tol-
erate higher doses of radiation and chemotherapeutic agents, pav-
ing the way for efforts to restrict exposure to bacteria for patients
receiving chemotherapy.[88] It was anticipated that protected environments and prophylactic antibiotics that reduced the incidence of infection would permit more intensive chemotherapy
for patients with acute leukemia.

Several types of isolation facilities have been used. The Life
Island includes a patient and bed surrounded by a plastic bubble.

The inflowing air is pumped through high-efficiency particulate-air (HEPA) filters that block particles larger than 0.3 μm in diameter. In the more complex and more expensive laminar air flow room (LAFR), one wall consists of HEPA filters. The flow of air is horizontal, in one direction, at 90 ft/minute. There is also a semiportable LAFR in which the velocity of air flow can be adjusted; it is usually set at 30 ft/minute.[88]

The first laminar air flow units for patients undergoing chemotherapy were installed at M. D. Anderson Cancer Center in 1967.[89] The widely accepted gut-sterilizing regimen of gentamicin, vancomycin, and nystatin was also introduced at our institution. Gentamicin and vancomycin were first used in 1967.[90]

Bodey et al. (1971) studied 33 patients with acute leukemia who underwent chemotherapy while also receiving antibiotics and residing under isolation in Life Island units or laminar air flow rooms. Two similar patients were considered as controls for each trial patient. "The complete remission rate was 61 percent for patients receiving the prophylactic program compared to 48 percent for control patients."[88] The durations of remission and survival were significantly longer for the protected persons, and the frequency of infection as related to the neutrophil count was significantly less.[90]

A report from the NCI (1973) citing the authors' prospective randomized study showed that patients with acute leukemia treated in a protected environment (isolation and air-filtration facilities) and given an extensive prophylactic antimicrobial regimen had approximately half as many severe infections and one quarter as many life-threatening infections as had patients treated conventionally. Among those who received only antibiotics or no prophylaxis, 22 to 24 percent died of infection during remission-induction therapy; no deaths from that cause occurred in the group treated with antibiotics in the protected environment.[91]

Although these early trials were for patients with acute leukemia, subsequent studies have featured other types of cancer. Fifty-eight patients with malignant lymphoma were randomly assigned to receive three courses of remission-induction chemotherapy on the protected environment-prophylactic antibiotic (PEPA) program (30 persons) or as controls (28 persons). Control patients received chemotherapy in the usual hospital room. The frequency of infection was significantly lower among those on the PEPA regime, and dosage of the chemotherapeutic agents was escalated more often. Dosage escalation did not increase the complete-remission rate, but it did reduce the relapse rate and significantly reduce the fatality rate. The durations of remission and survival were significantly longer for those patients whose dosage could be escalated.[92]

Bodey et al. (1981) reported a controlled trial in which 51 patients with malignant sarcomas were randomly allocated to receive three courses of remission-induction chemotherapy on the PEPA program (24) or as controls (27). The complete-remission rate was 33 percent for the PEPA group and 15 percent for the control cohort. The frequency of infection was significantly lower in the PEPA group and doses of chemotherapy could be escalated more often, resulting in a higher complete-remission rate and a lower fatality rate.[93]

In a recent (1987) article, Hortobagyi et al. described an induction chemotherapy trial for metastatic breast cancer in which patients were randomly assigned to laminar air flow rooms and prophylactic antibiotic treatment or to regular hospital rooms. Overall and complete-response rates were not significantly different, nor were times to progression or survival between the two groups.[94]

Bodey believes that the protected environment/prophylactic antibiotic arrangement has achieved the original objective: it has reduced the risk of infection and allowed the use of higher doses of chemotherapy. Unfortunately, "the more intensive chemotherapy only minimally improved response rates or durations of response."[95]

Although controversy exists,[96,97] the laminar air flow unit has been accepted as a supportive measure. Advances in cancer chemotherapy and in antibiotic therapy have occurred since the 1970s, when many of the controlled trials were initiated. Additional studies are needed to evaluate the current status of this prophylactic approach.

BONE MARROW TRANSPLANTATION

By 1936, Osgood and Muscovitz, at the University of Oregon Medical School, had developed a simple technique for obtaining human bone marrow during life by sternal puncture. Subsequently, they outlined their ambitious program to (1) isolate each type of cell in pure culture and determine the origin of each; (2) seek specific stimuli that would cause multiplication, maturation, or metaplasia; (3) determine characteristics in marrow from persons of different ages and sexes and those having various blood dyscrasias; (4) observe whether adding carcinogenic agents would produce leukemic changes in marrow cultures; (5) evaluate the effects of deficiencies of hormones, vitamins, minerals, and amino acids on growth and maturation of normal and diseased marrows; (6) record the effects of benzene, radium, x-rays, bacteria, and other agents; (7) test whether antibodies are formed by marrow cells and by which cell type; (8) determine the ingredients essential for the formation of hemoglobin; and (9) attempt to grow pure cultures of neutrophilic leukocytes for transfusion during infection. These might even be immunized by vaccines of the particular organism.[98] Of course, all of these goals were not accomplished, but the authors' aspirations must be admired.

In 1938, Osgood published his standardized nomenclature for cells of blood and marrow so that differential cell counts made in one laboratory could be compared with those in another. He also presented a table for cell identification to guide an observer in identifying a cell under the microscope, even though such a cell had never been heard of or seen before.[99]

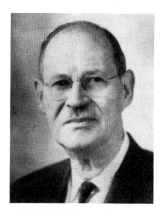

Osgood et al. (1939) cited a case history of a patient with aplastic anemia who lived 53 days after admission to the hospital in extremis. She received 43 blood transfusions, totaling 21,870 ml of blood, and sternal bone marrow (obtained from her brother, a compatible donor) was administered

Edwin E. Osgood

intravenously with no effect. The authors believed that the intravenous marrow infusion would eventually "take," but the woman succumbed to infection. They had attempted previously to inject bone marrow intrasternally, but, for technical reasons, they were unable to accomplish this.[100]

To Morrison and Samwick (1940), introducing bone marrow intrasternally was a simple matter. They commented, "One is surprised with the ease with which the contents are expelled from the syringe with only the slightest amount of pressure."[101] They treated a patient suffering from idiopathic aplastic anemia and believed that an unknown component present in normal marrow might stimulate maturation of hematopoietic constituents already present in the diseased marrow, thus supplying a factor to overcome a deficiency disease. In leukemia, this unknown deficient substance could allow the normal conversion of the myeloblast into a polymorphonuclear leukocyte. In granulocytopenia the myeloblasts might be stimulated to function properly. The patient was given three sternal marrow injections, 3 ml and 5 ml from his brother and 5 ml from another donor. One or 2 days later, platelets began to appear on blood smears, and, at the same time, the bleeding tendency was less apparent. The white blood cell count had risen from a low of 750 to 4,300 at the 15th day and to 7,000 by 40 days. Bleeding had stopped.[101]

By the early 1950s, bone marrow transplantation had been shown to prevent the death of animals exposed to supralethal x-irradiation.[102] Lorenz et al.[103] stated that Rekers (1948)[104] had injected bone marrow into dogs after exposing them to 3.5-Gy radiation. However, the dogs' survival rates improved only equivocally.[103] In their own experiments, Lorenz and colleagues injected bone marrow into mice (either intravenously or intraperitoneally) postirradiation (9 Gy) and reported that it gave excellent protection from the acute irradiation syndrome. Twenty-six control animals died with severe leukopenia. Guinea pigs also benefit from intravenous bone marrow injection after irradiation.[103]

The clinical application of bone marrow transplantation soon followed. Between 1959 and 1962, 154 reports of these procedures appeared in the medical literature.[102] Thomas et al. reported results of intravenous marrow transfusions in five patients who received radiation or cytotoxic drugs for malignancies and in one patient with cerebral hemorrhage. A temporary graft occurred in one patient. Donors had been matched for ABO blood group only.[105] Mathé and associates[106] in Paris achieved temporary grafts of marrow from ABO-compatible donors in five recipients who had been exposed accidentally to lethal radiation.[107] In general, the results of these early transplantations were very poor, and relatively few cases were reported between 1962 and 1970.[102]

During 1968 and 1969, however, several successful transplantations in infants were reported, which created renewed interest in the procedure. Bach (1968) reported that a 2-year-old boy with Wiskott-Aldrich syndrome was given a 4-day course of cyclophosphamide followed by bone marrow transplanted from a sister who was HLA-identical. Six weeks later, the boy showed no evidence of graft-versus-host disease and was doing well clinically.[108] Gatti and associates (1968)[109] and DeKoning et al. (1969)[110] reported successful bone marrow transplantations in 5-month-old boys who had lymphopenic immunologic deficiencies. In both cases, the donors were HLA-compatible siblings.

By the early 1970s, physicians were achieving successful results with the majority of initial allogeneic bone marrow transplantations. They had also learned a great deal about graft-versus-host problems. When genetically nonidentical tissue is transferred to a recipient, a reaction occurs, especially if the tissue is rich in immunologically competent cells. Such tissues include spleen, lymph nodes, thoracic duct lymph, and, to a lesser degree, the bone marrow and peripheral blood. The graft may not be rejected if the recipient is immunologically immature (e.g., newborn), if the recipient is a victim of certain immune-deficiency disorders, or if the recipient has received whole-body irradiation or an immunosuppressive agent. Graft-versus-host disease primarily affects the skin, gastrointestinal tract, and liver; the disorder may follow an acute or a chronic pattern.

In 1975, Thomas and colleagues wrote that 33 of 34 grafts in patients with aplastic anemia and 63 of 68 in patients with acute leukemia were successful.[111] They had prepared recipients with a modification of the regimen developed by Santos,[112] which required 50 mg of cyclophosphamide per kg of body weight on each of 4 days, followed 36 hours later by the marrow infusion. Thomas and associates administered the cyclophosphamide 24 hours after infusing antigen from the prospective donor, usually in the form of buffy coat cells.[113]

Thomas et al. (1977) performed bone marrow transplantations in 100 patients considered to be in the end stages of acute leu-

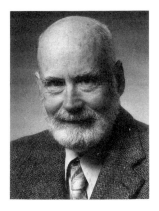

E. Donnall Thomas

kemia because of maximum chemo-therapy exposure, repeated relapses, or refractory central nervous system disease. Ninety of these persons were in relapse at the time of transplantation. After receiving chemotherapy and 10-Gy total-body irradiation, all were given a marrow graft from an HLA-identical sibling. Six patients died 3 to 17 days after marrow infusion without evidence of engraftment; only 1 patient rejected the graft. Thirteen persons were alive with no maintenance antileukemic therapy and without recurrent leukemia 1 to 4½ years after transplantation. Fifty persons developed moderate to severe graft-versus-host disease, and they were very susceptible to interstitial pneumonia, most often caused by cytomegalovirus. Thirty-one persons suffered a relapse of leukemia. Patients in fair clinical condition at the time of transplantation survived significantly longer than those in poor condition.[114]

As a result of the work of Thomas et al. and others, which showed that patients in good clinical and hematologic condition have a better graft prognosis, studies of allogeneic bone marrow transplantation for patients in early stages of acute leukemia soon followed. Those with acute myeloblastic leukemia who achieved a first remission with combination chemotherapy were facing a median survival of 12 to 15 months. Therefore, it was deemed ethically acceptable to consider early transplantation,[115] and the Seattle team initiated it. Nineteen patients with ANLL in first remission were prepared with cyclophosphamide and total-body irradiation (9.2 Gy) and infused with marrow from HLA-identical siblings. Ten of 19 were alive and in remission 5 to 7 years after grafting.[115,116] Today, physicians at some cancer centers advocate bone marrow transplantation during the first complete remission, but those at other centers are reluctant because of the high morbidity and mortality resulting from complications of the procedure.

When a patient who has newly diagnosed acute leukemia

achieves a first remission with induction chemotherapy, is it better to advise marrow transplantation (if a donor is available) or to continue chemotherapy? Appelbaum and colleagues (1984), with the Seattle group, compared 44 adults who had acute nonlymphoblastic leukemia in first remission and had donors available with 46 similar patients without matched donors. Thirty-three of 44 in the former group received transplantations; all 46 in the latter cohort continued to receive chemotherapy. Kaplan-Meier estimates of 5-year disease-free survival rates from the time of complete remission were 49 percent (± 18 percent) for the transplanted group and 20 percent (± 13 percent) for the chemotherapy group. Transplantation recipients had a higher risk of dying during the first 6 months after remission induction but a lower risk of dying thereafter. Age was the only factor significantly influencing survival in the transplantation group.[117]

An analogous comparison at M. D. Anderson Cancer Center (1988) showed that patients who received transplants had significantly better control of leukemia; however, survival duration was improved only in the poor- and intermediate-risk groups.[118] A report of a similar trial by Los Angeles investigators revealed that bone marrow transplantation is more effective than continued chemotherapy in preventing relapse but does not improve overall survival rate.[119]

The earliest report of marrow transfusion in patients with CML may be that of Buckner et al. (1974). Two persons in blastic transformation were given supralethal doses of total-body irradiation followed by autologous marrow infusion. One patient achieved engraftment of myeloid, erythroid, and megakaryotic elements but not lymphoid elements and died of cardiopulmonary complications 83 days after marrow infusion. The second patient had incomplete engraftment and died of infection 48 days after marrow infusion.[120]

In 1924, Minot and colleagues reported that patients with CML lived an average of 3 years after noticing the first symptom and an average of 1.6 years after diagnosis.[121] Today, the median survival from diagnosis is usually reported. "During the past 50 years, treatment of CGL has consisted mainly of palliative measures with busulfan, hydroxyurea, or splenectomy. The median survival from diagnosis, however, remains 2 to 4 years, with less than 20% of patients surviving 5 years and with no cures."[122]

Fefer et al. (1986) presented a retrospective analysis of patients with Ph[1]-positive CGL who, between April 1970 and November 1984, received marrow transplantations from HLA-matched siblings in Seattle. At the time of transplantation, 23 persons were in blastic phase, 33 were in accelerated phase, and 45 were in chronic phase. After a follow-up of 1 to 8 years, the probability of long-term survival was 14 percent (blastic), 10 percent (accelerated), and 58 percent (chronic). Patients <30 years old who are in the chronic phase have a 70 percent probability of long-term survival. Patients >30 years old show an increased incidence of transplant-related complications, especially graft-versus-host disease and interstitial pneumonitis. Three of 23 in the blastic, 8 of 33 in the accelerated, and 29 of 45 in the chronic phase survived.[122]

Also in 1986, Fefer et al. reported that 16 patients in the chronic phase of Ph[1]-positive CGL received marrow transplanted from identical twins. Two died of pneumonitis, 3 continued to have CGL, and 11 remained in complete hematologic and cytogenetic remission without any Ph[1] metaphases at 31 to 108 months after transplantation. Thus, the Ph[1]-positive clone can be eradicated and blast crisis prevented.[123]

Age is an important factor in successful bone marrow transplantation. In a recent cooperative study of patients with CML,[124] the rate of long-term survival with a potential of cure was over 80 percent in patients younger than 25 years but only slightly over 50 percent in patients above that age. The results were similar for persons with acute leukemia. Speck stated that grafts are hardly ever successful in patients older than 40,[125] and investigators from the Seattle team wrote, "For patients more than 50 years of age, allogeneic marrow grafting cannot presently be considered first-line therapy."[126]

Barnes et al. (1956)[127] were the first to show that leukemic mice subjected to total-body irradiation and syngeneic bone marrow transplantation died with leukemia, whereas those transplanted with allogeneic marrow died with graft-versus-host disease with no indications of leukemia.[128] These results were later confirmed in other animal laboratories.

In 1965, Mathé et al. wrote that graft-versus-host disease might be used against tumors. They coined the term *adoptive immunotherapy*,[129] writing that "the theoretical principle of treatment of acute leukemia by adoptive immunotherapy is to permit allogeneic, immunologically competent cells to act against the host's leukemic cells and the basic leukemogenic factors present in the host."[129] They believed that, if the patient survived the secondary syndrome induced by the graft, the leukemia might be eradicated. They described their treatment of spontaneous, transplanted, and viral leukemias in mice and also clinical trials in humans.

Weiden et al. (1979) reported outcomes of studies designed to determine whether allogeneic bone marrow transplantation is associated with a graft-versus-leukemia effect. They examined the relationship between the occurrence of graft-versus-host disease and leukemia relapse by comparing 46 recipients of identical-twin (syngeneic) marrow, 117 recipients of HLA-identical sibling (allogeneic) marrow with no or minimal graft-versus-host disease, and 79 recipients of allogeneic marrow with moderate to severe or chronic disease. The relative relapse rate was 2.5 times less for allogeneic-marrow recipients with graft-versus-host disease than for recipients without it. However, the survivals of all patients were comparable because the lesser probability of recurrent leukemia in patients with graft-versus-host disease was offset by a greater probability of death from other causes.[130]

Gale and Champlin (1984) studied patients who had AML in first remission. The relapse rate was 59 percent (± 20 percent) in 31 recipients of identical-twin transplantations, whereas it was 18 percent (± 4 percent) in 339 recipients of HLA-identical sibling grafts.[131,132] A similar study from the International Bone Marrow Transplant Registry (1985) also indicated an increased risk of relapse in patients who received marrow from a twin (65 percent [± 24 percent] versus 20 percent [± 7 percent]).[132,133]

Gale and Champlin stated:

> Bone marrow transplantation from an HLA-identical sibling is effective in eradicating leukaemia in most patients with AML in first remission. The efficacy is widely assumed to be related to the high doses of drugs and radiation administered before transplantation. . . . However, in animals there is considerable evidence that the antileukaemic efficacy of bone marrow transplantation is partly due to a graft-versus-leukaemia reaction.[131]

Fefer et al. from the Seattle team analyzed all of their patients undergoing bone marrow transplantation between 1970 and 1986. Leukemia recurred in 62 percent of 785 allogeneic recipients and in 75 percent of 53 syngeneic recipients (P <0.0001). These figures tend to support a graft-versus-leukemia effect from allogeneic marrow.[128]

Autologous Bone Marrow Transplantation (ABMT)

Because the majority of patients who have leukemia do not have an available HLA-identical donor and also because of the possibility of graft-versus-host disease, many physicians turned to ABMT, a procedure presenting no immunologic obstacles. In addition, it meets the needs of older patients.

As mentioned previously, Thomas and colleagues (1957)[105] had tried intravenous infusion of bone marrow from donors matched for ABO blood group only. Because there were problems with the grafts "taking" and because delayed deaths were attributed to antibody production, either from the host against the graft or from the grafted tissue against the host, Kurnick et al. (1958) thought that these difficulties might be avoided with autogenous bone marrow. They limited their patients to those in whom malignant disease had not involved the bone marrow, noting that "the effect of administering autogenous leukemic marrow to a heavily irradiated patient cannot be predicted."[134] Their first patient suffered from metastatic testicular carcinoma, and the second had an almost terminal case of renal carcinoma with pulmonary metastases. Both received irradiation to the entire torso, after which stored marrow was infused. The first man improved somewhat for about a month and then succumbed to extensive metastatic disease; the second died soon after infusion. The authors concluded: "Because of the severe hematopoietic depression which results from rapid, intensive irradiation of the thoracolumbar region, potentially curable malignancies are often inadequately irradiated. The likelihood of salvaging such . . . cases would be considerably enhanced if irradiation could be pursued with less concern for the ensuing hematopoietic depression."[134]

In another early publication concerning ABMT (1959), Mc-Govern et al. wrote that, "during a remission of acute leukemia in children induced by one of the chemotherapeutic agents, the bone marrow may return temporarily to a normal morphologic state. Thus, the question arises whether in some cases the marrow may provide an acceptable source of autologous material for subsequent use as a marrow autograft."[135] These investigators stored marrow taken during remission and infused it later after the patient had received a potentially lethal dose of total-body irradiation during a period of critical relapse. Their first three patients were young children who had acute lymphoblastic leukemia. The first died 9 days after irradiation with leukemia still present, and the third died 23 days after irradiation with no evidence of leukemia or repopulation of bone marrow. However, the second child (2 years old) recovered normal marrow within 17 days and entered a clinical and hematologic remission.[135]

Physicians gave little attention to ABMT until the late 1970s, after allogeneic transplantation had been expanded. By that time, techniques for successfully cryopreserving bone marrow stem cells had been developed, and the thawed marrow had been proved to present no undue danger to recipients. By 1978, scattered reports of ABMT in a few patients with acute leukemia appeared in the literature, and, in 1979, results of a sizable group study were published by Dicke and associates at M. D. Anderson Cancer Center.

Twenty-one evaluable patients with acute leukemia in irreversible relapse were given high-dose piperazinedione and supralethal total-body irradiation in conjunction with ABMT. Eleven achieved complete remissions; all of these had had the bone marrow aspirated during the first remission. Nineteen of 21 had evidence of engraftment, but 7 died before achieving complete remission.[136]

Although the marrow is aspirated from the patient during a remission, tumor cells in varying amounts are usually present, and diverse methods for purging the marrow have been tried. In vivo purging occurs when the patient receives remission-induction chemotherapy and, after his marrow regenerates, a supply is removed for later use after high-dose intensification chemotherapy. Ex vivo purging has been accomplished with many different drugs (some in concentrations not achievable in vivo) and also with monoclonal antibodies. As Horwitz and colleagues explained:

A number of novel approaches to purging bone marrow have been tried. Most of these are still too early to determine the clinical anti-leukemic effect. However, on the basis of inversion rates and long-term survival, there seems to be promise in AML with *ex vivo* chemotherapy and in ALL using monoclonal antibody pools. Using combinations of modalities, combinations of drugs *ex vivo*, or novel ways of separating cells may prove to be even more effective approaches in eradicating leukemia cells.[137]

Santos and Colvin (1986) listed their requirements for an ideal agent to be used for marrow purging:

1. demonstrates that it does not have severe hematopoietic stem cell toxicity as its limiting toxicity when used in vivo;
2. is employable ex vivo at a concentration exceeding the maximally tolerated in vivo concentration by at least several fold;
3. demonstrates greater differential sensitivity of the clonogenic tumor cell than of the hematopoietic stem cell;
4. is able to kill tumor cells independent of cell cycle;
5. is easy to use ex vivo and able to be inactivated or eliminated before or diluted to nontoxic levels with the infusion of the treated marrow;
6. is noncarcinogenic to normal cells not eliminated by the purging procedure.[138]

In 1987, Dicke et al. reported the use of high-dose cytoreductive programs in conjunction with ABMT to treat 127 patients who had acute leukemia. Transplantation during relapse resulted in complete-remission rates ranging from 33 to 72 percent, depending on the time of transplantation, the conditioning regimen used, and the performance status of the patient. Remission durations were short, varying from 3 to 9 months. Transplantation in second or subsequent remission did not change the natural history of the disease. Transplantation in first remission resulted in a projected 2-year disease-free survival rate of 72 percent for patients with AML and of 45 percent for those with ALL.[139]

Bortin and Rimm (1986) found that 2,500 persons underwent bone marrow transplantation (of all types) in 1985. About 9,500 transplantations occurred from 1958 through 1984. In the years before 1980, 72 percent of the transplantations reported to the International Bone Marrow Transplant Registry were for non-malignant diseases, but, since 1980, 77 percent have been for malignancies.[140]

E. Donnall Thomas was a co-recipient of the Nobel Prize in medicine for 1990 in recognition of his many contributions to the collective knowledge of transplantation.

SEVEN

Biologic Response Modifiers

Natural forces within us are the
true healers of disease.

HIPPOCRATES (460–377 B.C.)

Dr. W. B. Coley, in 1891, may have been the first to report the use of biologic agents to treat cancer. He described remarkable results using bacterial cell filtrates and sometimes administering *Streptococcus erysipelatis* by scarification or injection to treat sarcoma.[1] Goldstein and Laszlo stated that his theories were not pursued because his therapy caused severe side effects and because modern cancer surgery and radiotherapy came to the forefront.[2]

The phrase *biologic response modifiers* (BRMs) was first introduced by Dr. Vincent T. DeVita, Jr., Director of the NCI, during a meeting addressing the problem of how to focus increased attention on basic biologic research.[3]

A committee on biologic response modifiers was appointed in 1978 at the NCI to study the available information on interferon and other products of living organisms that might have an effect on cancer. As a result of a 2-year investigation into the future of this area of research, $13.5 million were allocated in 1980 to launch a BRM program. The primary goal was to create a working plan for promoting and coordinating research with biologic response modifiers. According to Oldham, the classes of agents to be investigated included "immuno-augmenting, immunomodulating and immunorestorative agents, interferons and interferon inducers, lymphokines, cytokines, antigrowth factors, thymic factors, tumor antigens and modifiers of tumor antigens on cell membranes, antitumor antibodies, antitumor cells, and maturation and differentiation factors."[4]

Biologic agents are naturally occurring proteins that act as messengers between cells. They are called *cytokines* because they originate in cells and are called *interleukins* when they function as messengers between leukocytes.[5]

In 1986, the NCI was screening approximately 10,000 possible cytotoxic agents in vivo each year, using P388 murine leukemia models.[6,7] More recently, the NCI has been shifting its emphasis to human cells for greater specificity against human tumors.[6,8] Screening of BRMs is more complicated than screening of chemotherapeutic agents. The latter destroy malignant cells, but BRMs are aimed at one or more classes of host activator cells, which are the intermediaries in a subsequent counteraction against the cancer.[6] The Biologic Response Modifiers Program Preclinical Screening Laboratory has each year evaluated the effects of 10 to 20 compounds on macrophage, natural-killer cell, and lymphocyte functions in tumor-free mice and on tumor growth in metastatic transplant and autochthonous murine tumor models.[6,9,10] As Hawkins et al. said, "because many cytotoxic agents may be toxic to effector cells, the addition of BRMs to existing chemotherapy regimens is conceptually complex. . . . there is no model that can be used to combine BRMs with cytotoxic chemotherapy in an optimal manner."[6]

We include here brief discussions of the more prominent BRMs that have been tested thus far.

BACILLUS CALMETTE-GUÉRIN (BCG) VACCINE

This substance was first developed by Calmette and Guérin at the Pasteur Institute in 1908 and was first used in France in 1921, when it was administered orally to a newborn who had a family member with active tuberculosis. The baby had no ill effects; he was monitored until he was 33 and did not develop tuberculosis.[11] Subsequently, many children, individually or included in several large studies, received the vaccine with varying results, but no controlled trials were conducted; investigators disagreed strongly regarding the effectiveness of BCG in preventing tuberculosis.[12] In 1930, a batch of vaccine prepared in a German laboratory was contaminated with live bacilli, causing 72 deaths in Lübeck and giving the vaccine a reputation for being dangerous.[11]

The first documented use of BCG in treating cancer was by Holmgren in 1935.[13] He gave 28 persons with cancer 185 i.v. injections with no serious untoward effects but also no spectacular improvements.[11,12] Twenty-four years later (1959), Halpern et al.[14] found that, "in animals, BCG stimulated immune reactivity in a nonspecific way and increased the animal's capacity to resist a subsequent challenge with bacteria or tumour."[15]

Also in 1959, Old and colleagues reported that, when mice received implants of sarcoma-180 1 day after being infected with BCG, the tumor regression rate was not affected. When mice were inoculated with the tumor 7 or more days after BCG infection, however, they showed definite protection. Tumors regressed in 70 to 75 percent of mice inoculated with sarcoma-180 7 to 19 days after receiving BCG; those inoculated with tumor 14, 25, and 67 days after receiving BCG were completely resistant to tumor growth.[16] The following year, the same group of researchers wrote that survival time increased twofold in BCG-infected hosts inoculated with Ehrlich ascites. They believed that BCG causes profound reticuloendothelial stimulation, enhances resistance to bacterial challenges, and increases the capacity of the host to form antibodies.[17]

During the 1960s, epidemiologic studies showed positive results for the vaccine in preventing leukemia. Immunization with BCG vaccine during the first 3 days of life (with the mother's consent) commenced in Austria in 1949. Since then, mortality from CML has declined from 7/100,000 to 2/100,000, and the researchers credit the immunization.[12] Ambrosch et al., referring to that same inoculation program, "found a reduction of the overall leukemia morbidity in vaccinated children by 34%. . . . a protective effect of BCG vaccination against leukemia is highly probable."[18]

From 1946 through 1949, a campaign was conducted in Finland for mass immunization with BCG vaccine. In a 1986 report, Härö presented some of the results. Male birth-year cohorts from 1926 through 1941 were analyzed, comparing observed with expected ratios of leukemia incidence. During the period 1949 through 1978, which was the follow-up interval, 422 cases of leukemia developed in these cohorts. Approximately 533,000 persons in the cohorts were studied, 315,000 of whom received BCG. About 115,000 were tuberculin positive, and about 200,000 were tuberculin negative and BCG vaccinated. There was no marked difference between the naturally tuberculosis-infected and the BCG-vaccinated persons. Participants had considerably fewer cases of leukemia than nonparticipants, a great many of whom were not vaccinated and not infected (see Table).[19]

Since 1955, all neonates in Israel, except for those born in Jerusalem, have been immunized. Observation of leukemia incidence has revealed a relative risk for children born in Jerusalem 1.5 times greater than that for children born elsewhere.[12]

In 1965, Villasor used BCG vaccine to treat 43 patients who had various types of advanced cancer. The treated patients' survival rate at 2 years was superior to that of the control group, who received only chemotherapy.[20]

Mathé and associates (1969) used scarification with BCG to prolong remissions in 20 patients with ALL after chemotherapy had induced a remission. Eight persons had not relapsed when the article was published; the longest remission at that time was 1,150 days. All 10 controls had relapsed.[21]

Davignon et al. (1970) found that, among children less than

Leukemia Incidence

Status	Number of Cases	
	Observed	*Expected*
Tuberculin −, BCG vaccinated	36	104
Tuberculin +	64	152
Nonparticipants	322	166
Total	422	422

SOURCE: Härö AS: The effect of BCG vaccination and tuberculosis on the risk of leukaemia. *Dev Biol Stand* 58(Part A):433–449, 1986
ABBREVIATION: BCG, bacillus Calmette-Guérin

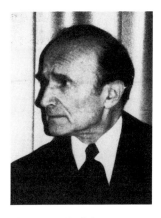

Georges Mathé

15 years old who lived in the province of Quebec, death from leukemia in each of the years 1960 to 1963 occurred half as often in those vaccinated with BCG as in those not vaccinated."

The Concord Trial (1971) dealt with 191 patients with ALL. They received chemotherapy for 5 months and then were randomized to receive BCG, twice-weekly methotrexate, or no further treatment. Complete remissions were achieved by 177 (93 percent). At 26 months, 143 were still living, including 70 in their first remission. Median remission lengths were 17 weeks (no treatment), 27 weeks (BCG), and 52 weeks (methotrexate).[23]

Soon after Mathé's report of patients with ALL, physicians began trying BCG against AML. Results of two early studies were very encouraging.[15,24] Powles and colleagues studied 45 patients who had AML and in whom chemotherapy had achieved a remission. All continued to receive chemotherapy for 5 of every 28 days. Group A (19 of 45) was given no other therapy and, when the article was written, 7 patients remained alive, only 5 still in first remission. Group B (23 of 45) received, in addition, immunotherapy consisting of multiple weekly intradermal injections of irradiated stored AML cells plus BCG administered with a Heaf gun. Sixteen persons of Group B remained alive, 8 still in first remission. The difference in survival rate is statistically significant. No mention was made of the outcome for the remaining 3 patients.[15]

Gutterman et al. (1974) described a trial involving 53 consecutive adults who had acute leukemia; 20 made up the study cohort and 33 served as controls. The study cohort received intermittent chemoimmunotherapy with cytarabine, vincristine, and prednisone (OAP) plus BCG by scarification; 11 of 20 (55 percent) remained in remission with an estimated median duration of 91 weeks. Control subjects received the same chemotherapy regimen but no BCG. Only 14 of 33 (42 percent) of this group remained in remission after a median duration of 50 weeks. However, immunotherapy's effect was significant only for patients who had AML.[24]

In 1975, Carswell and colleagues found that the serum of BCG-infected mice treated with endotoxin contains a substance (tumor-necrosis factor) that mimics the tumor-necrotic action of endotoxin itself. Tests indicated that it is a factor released by host cells, probably macrophages.[25]

BCG is considered to be an immunoaugmenting agent and, when it is used in cancer therapy, multiple vaccinations may be given over a relatively short period. As Crispen wrote: "It is not unusual for a cancer patient to receive 25 or more vaccinations per year. This can lead to serious side effects ranging from anaphylaxis to death or to anergy."[11]

Over the years, BCG has been administered by about every possible route (oral, subcutaneous, intradermal, intramuscular, and intraperitoneal) and also by multiple puncture, scarification, atomizer, and nebulizer.[11] Of the many clinical trials using BCG since the early ones, some have shown positive results and others have shown no effect. The prognostic value of reactivity to BCG has been shown to be important in patients with malignant melanoma (Cachran et al., 1981)[26] and metastatic breast cancer (Hortobagyi et al., 1986).[27] Although BCG did not attain prominence as a therapy for leukemia, its contribution is important historically. It was the forerunner for later BRMs and the herald of immunotherapy.

According to DeVita (1982): "The power of the immunobiological data available to us today should clearly bring home the reason why nonspecific immunotherapy with materials like BCG was doomed to failure. The immunological system, as we know it, is too complex to be stimulated nonspecifically with the expectation of a single defined positive antitumor effect."[28]

INTERFERON

In recent years, researchers have detected and isolated substances that control or guide or regulate particular processes in healthy normal organisms. Interferon is one of these natural "regulators," and it was a welcome addition to the armamentarium against cancer because everyone hoped that it would be efficacious without having the devastating side effects of the chemotherapy agents.

According to Shorter (1987), in July 1956 Jean Lindenmann traveled from Zurich to London to spend a research year with virus specialist Alick Isaacs at the National Institute for Medical Research. In August, the two "have tea together . . . and discuss a curious phenomenon: once a person is infected by one kind of virus, he almost never comes down with a second viral disease simultaneously."[29] This is called *viral interference*. Aroused by the initial virus, the body must secrete something that protects against viruses.

By November 1956, the two scientists had found the unknown factor and named it *interferon*.

> During a study of the interference produced by heat-activated influenza virus with the growth of live virus in fragments of chick chorio-allantoic membrane, it was found that following incubation of heated virus with membrane, a new factor was released. This factor, recognized by its ability to induce interference in fresh pieces of chorio-allantoic membrane, was called interferon.[30]

> Interferons are proteins that are able to influence protoplasm in some way, rendering it resistant to virus infection. This consequence is apparent both in vitro and in vivo. The interferons constitute a very complicated group comprising numerous categories of proteins that act in a hormone-like manner.[31] It is possible that they stimulate cells to create their own defensive proteins, so that when a virus enters it is blocked, unable to reproduce further or exit.[29]

In 1959, a committee was organized in the United Kingdom to conduct experiments on interferon with the goal of progressing toward trials in humans. The committee included representatives from the research laboratories of several large pharmaceutical companies and members of the Medical Research Council. Three years later they reported that human interferon had been concentrated and purified and that standards of safety had been outlined. Interferon preparation from monkey kidney tissue had been inoculated intradermally into human volunteers who were vaccinated the next day with smallpox vaccine. Interferon prevented or reduced the size of the vaccinia lesions.[32]

A few years after the discovery of interferon, Atanasiu and Chany (1960)[33] presented evidence indicating that treating hamsters with a crude interferon preparation 16 to 24 hours before inoculating them with polyoma virus delayed the appearance of tumors, decreased the number of animals that developed tumors, and increased the length of survivals.[34] Allison (1961)[35] reported that interferon preparations suppressed oncogenic virus proliferation and also inhibited the cellular changes induced by these viruses.[34] During the 1960s, work on the production of interferon continued and treatment trials in lower animals were undertaken.

Investigators learned that, because of marked species specificity, interferon preparations to be used in humans must be prepared in primate cells[36] and that leukocytes are excellent producers of interferon. Although all existing human interferons may not yet have been found, 20 have been identified thus far.[2] They fall into at least three types: alpha-leukocyte, beta-fibroblast, and gamma-immune. Sixteen genes are now recognized as coding for alpha-interferon and have been assigned to chromosome 9.[31,37] Data indicate that beta-interferon genes are present on at least three different human chromosomes.[37]

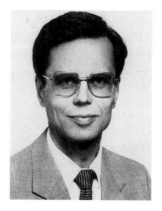

Kari Cantell

According to Shorter:

> In 1963, the Finnish virus specialist Kari Cantell of Helsinki's Central Public Health Laboratory dedicated himself to making available a small supply of interferon, extracted from donated blood. . . . But the amounts Cantell could derive were tiny. From 45,000 liters of blood he was able to extract only 400 mg of interferon—about one one-hundredth of an ounce. And even that tiny amount was only 1 percent pure, the other 99 percent of the solution he shipped out to various researchers

being other white-cell proteins, so it was impossible to get an interferon pure enough even to analyze its chemical composition.[29]

An article in *Time* magazine reported that, for therapeutic use, a pound of interferon at that time would have cost between $10 and $20 billion.[29,38]

The groundwork in preparing interferons for clinical use in cancer was necessarily slow because of their complexity and because they represented an entirely new classification of agents with a whole different array of biologic effects.[31] According to Kirkwood and Ernstoff[31] the use of alpha-interferon to treat human leukemia originated in France (1966),[39] but the most noteworthy and highly publicized work was that of Strander, Cantell, and colleagues in Sweden.

In 1973, Strander, Cantell, and Carlström reported a trial of 11 patients with malignant tumors (Hodgkin's disease, multiple myeloma, sarcoma, malignant melanoma, or cervical carcinoma in situ) who were given intramuscular injections of interferon three times weekly. Three of the patients also had herpes zoster, and all three experienced relief of pain and developed crusts within 1 week after beginning therapy. All 11 persons developed fevers and increased sedimentation rates, but none experienced serious side effects during treatment, which lasted >150 days in 3 cases. No definite antitumor effect was seen.[36]

At a workshop at Lake Placid, New York, in May 1973, Strander and Cantell, who had been administering intramuscular human leukocyte interferon to cancer patients at Karolinska Hospital, Stockholm, expressed the opinion that "an evaluation of exogenous interferon therapy against human neoplastic disease seems warranted."[40] They considered osteogenic sarcoma, Hodgkin's disease, and acute leukemia to be suitable candidates for study because a 1972 report had stated that all of them could be caused by the same virus.[41]

The following year (1974), Strander presented a paper at a conference sponsored by the Virus Cancer Program of the NCI. At Karolinska Hospital, 13 patients with osteogenic sarcoma had been treated with partially purified interferon administered intramuscularly. Ten of 13 had been monitored for more than 6 months, during which time none had developed pulmonary metastasis; in contrast, metastases had developed in 10 of 22 similar patients used as controls. No patient receiving interferon developed a serious side effect.[42]

The Wadley Institute of Molecular Medicine in Dallas started producing human leukocyte interferon in March 1976, and a year later Hill and colleagues began clinical trials with cancer patients. In 1981, they reported objective benefit in two of three patients with AML and in five of five patients with ALL when treated with high-dose interferon administered intravenously.[43]

About the same time Gutterman and associates (1982), reporting a trial of interferon, wrote:

> Recent progress in recombinant DNA technology and production of monoclonal antibodies has yielded a single purified species of leukocyte interferon. This study is the first clinical investigation of a purified recombinant-DNA-produced interferon; previous clinical studies of interferons have used preparations of approximately 1% purity. We know that these preparations contained a mixture of eight or more species of leukocyte interferon.[44]

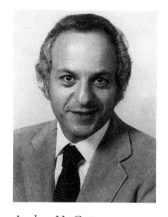

Gutterman and colleagues administered intramuscular interferon injections to 16 patients with advanced cancer (lymphocytic lymphoma, multiple myeloma, adenocarcinoma of breast or ovary, or CML). Side effects included fever, chills, myalgia, headache, fatigue, and reversible leukopenia and granulocytopenia, and 8 patients reported transient and mild numbness of hands, feet, or both. Seven of the 16 persons showed objective evidence of tumor regression.[44]

Jordan U. Gutterman

Also in 1982, Hersh et al. characterized the host defense factors and prognosis of patients with hairy cell leukemia.[45] During that period at M. D. Anderson, the majority of these patients were dying of bone marrow failure and subsequent infection within 1 month to 2 years after diagnosis.[46] In 1984, Quesada and colleagues from the same institution treated

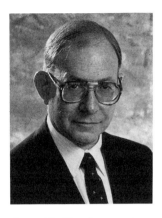

Evan M. Hersh

seven patients who had progressive hairy cell leukemia with partially pure alpha (leukocyte) interferon. Three persons achieved complete remissions and four had partial remissions, according to very strict criteria for response. Alpha-interferon seemed to be highly effective against hairy cell leukemia.[47]

By 1986, Quesada, Hersh, and associates wrote that they had used recombinant alpha-interferon to treat 30 patients who had hairy cell leukemia, 7 of whom had not been treated previously. Bone marrow core biopsies documented 9 complete and 17 partial remissions. Seven persons had splenomegaly, and in all the spleen promptly shrank to normal size. The incidence of complete remissions was significantly higher for previously untreated persons (5 of 7) than for those who had had splenectomy (4 of 23).[48]

In June 1986, the FDA approved the use of two synthetic alpha-interferon products to treat hairy cell leukemia; a 90 percent remission rate influenced or prompted this approval.[49] In 1984, Spiers and colleagues reported and other investigators confirmed that pentostatin was highly effective against hairy cell leukemia.[50] Controlled trials comparing interferon to pentostatin are currently in progress.[51,52]

Alpha-interferon has also proven to be of value against CML. In 1983, Talpaz and associates treated seven patients who had CML with partially purified human leukocyte interferon, 9 to 15 $\times$ 10^6 units daily by intramuscular injection. Five (70 percent) achieved hematologic remissions and, in about 20 percent of the recipients, the Ph^1 chromosome was completely or partially eliminated.[5,53]

In 1986, when recombinant interferon became available, Talpaz et al. treated 17 persons who had Ph^1-positive CML with 5 $\times$ 10^6 units/sq m/day intramuscularly. Thirteen patients attained a complete hematologic remission and one had a partial hematologic remission. All therapy was given on an outpatient basis, and no patient required hospitalization because of complications;

side effects included fatigue, depression, and insomnia. Five persons had complete cytogenetic suppression, which has lasted up to 3½ years in all except one.[54]

A year later Talpaz et al. (1987) reported that 51 patients with previously untreated or minimally treated CML in the chronic phase had received alpha-interferon daily, 3 to 9×10^6 units intramuscularly, until they achieved a complete hematologic remission. They were then maintained at lower or similar doses every other day. Forty-one (80 percent) responded, and 36 (71 percent) attained complete remissions. The Ph^1 chromosome was suppressed in 20 of the 36 in complete remission after a median of 9 months' therapy. After a median follow-up period of 37 months, disease in 25 patients remained controlled with interferon. Acute toxic reactions were moderate. Chronic toxicities (skeletal, muscular, and joint pains; neurotoxicity; immune-mediated thrombocytopenia) were treatment-limiting in 12 percent of the patients.[55]

The same group of clinicians reported hopeful results using recombinant gamma-interferon, 0.25 to 0.50 mg/sq m/day intramuscularly, in patients with Ph^1-positive benign-phase CML. Twenty-six of 30 patients were evaluable; 6 achieved a complete and 4 a partial hematologic response. No relapses have occurred among complete responders during a median follow-up period of 7.5 months. Five persons had cytogenetic improvement. The authors have now started therapeutic trials using combination interferon therapy.[56]

In a review article, Gutterman summarized, "Interferon-α is essentially inactive in CML in blast crisis and only modestly effective during the accelerated phase, but it is extremely effective in the chronic phase."[5]

INTERLEUKIN 2 (IL-2)

As mentioned in chapter 2, Morgan et al. (1976) showed that T lymphocytes secrete a protein that sustains the proliferation of T cells. The protein was termed *T cell growth factor*[57] and subsequently renamed *interleukin 2*. T cells are thymus-derived cells that play a major role in the immune reaction; they are involved in cell-mediated responses to foreign antigens. Investigators later learned that simply introducing IL-2 does not cause the T cells to begin proliferating. First, they must be presented with a precisely prepared antigen from protoplasm that has been consumed by a macrophage.[58] Surface receptors for IL-2 then appear on the T cells, and IL-2 stimulates the T cells to multiply. However, recent publications have presented evidence that resting T cells, not under antigenic stimulation, may also be induced by IL 2 to proliferate and to accomplish other functions.[59,60] In 1986 Lifson et al. stated that "the capacity to induce this response [proliferation] is a property of the IL-2 molecule itself."[59]

Interleukin 2 is a *lymphokine,* which is a general term for factors released by sensitized lymphocytes on contact with an antigen. Interleukins are a special variety of lymphokine that activate other lymphocytes. Monocytes secrete interleukin 1, which stimulates T lymphocytes to produce IL-2. The gene for IL-2 has been cloned,[60–62] and its location on human chromosome 4 has been reported.[60,63]

IL-2 supports the growth of human cytotoxic T cells, induces antigen-specific T cell lines to produce B cell growth factor, enhances gamma-interferon production,[64] and also stimulates the production of distinctive lymphocytes called natural killer (NK) cells, which are considered to be tumoricidal. Lotze et al. (NCI, 1981) reported lysis of fresh and cultured autologous tumor by human lymphocytes cultured in T cell growth factor (IL-2).[65] This lysis also occurred with NK cell-resistant tumor cell lines, so these special lymphocytes were called lymphokine-activated killer (LAK) cells.

After small trials of LAK cells alone and IL-2 alone in humans proved to be ineffective, Rosenberg, Lotze, and colleagues (1985) reported results of a trial using the two combined in 25 patients with advanced metastatic cancer; cancer regressed more than 50 percent in 11 of these 25 persons. Therapy with combined LAK cells and IL-2 produced positive results in patients for whom no adequate treatment had been available. Significant fluid retention was the major side effect.[66] The article was published in the *New England Journal of Medicine* and was immediately heralded in the lay media. The cover of *Fortune* for November 25, 1985, featured two vials of IL-2 with CANCER BREAKTHROUGH printed as a bold head.[58] Patients with cancer, their families, and their physicians were vociferous in clamoring for supplies of the miracle medicine. The outcry brought back memories of the commotion triggered by the debut of interferon.

In December 1986, in the *Journal of the American Medical Association*, Lotze et al. (NCI) reported results of high-dose re-combinant IL-2 therapy for 10 patients with disseminated cancer. Disease regressed in 3 of 6 who had melanoma, but none of 4 persons with colorectal or ovarian cancer responded. Responses lasted 1, 3, and 7 months without further treatment.[67] In an editorial in the same issue of *JAMA*, Moertel (Mayo Clinic) criticized therapy with IL-2 because of its "unacceptably severe toxicity and astronomical costs" without any "persuasive evidence of true net therapeutic gain."[68,69]

In 1987, Pui et al. measured serum IL-2 receptor levels in 59 children with non-Hodgkin's lymphoma and in 6 children with B cell ALL and confirmed that those with the highest levels were more likely to fail treatment. In the past, the most reliable prognostic factors for childhood non-Hodgkin's lymphoma were the stage of disease at the time of diagnosis and the serum lactic dehydrogenase level. However, the soluble IL-2 receptor level was found to have greater predictive strength than either of these.[70]

Jermy and associates (1987) showed that NK cell activity was severely reduced in children undergoing maintenance chemo-therapy for ALL.[71] They investigated the ability of IL-2 to enhance the spontaneous NK activity of peripheral-blood lymphocytes, using samples of blood from 42 children with ALL and 8 child controls. IL-2 pretreatment augmented the NK cell activity of the peripheral-blood lymphocytes from all 8 control subjects, but only 24 of the 42 samples from children with ALL showed increased activity.[72]

In a phase II trial, Allison and colleagues (1989) administered IL-2 at 1 mg/sq m to 18 patients and at 0.5 mg/sq m to 17 patients for 5 days every other week for a total of 8 weeks. Persons who had malignant lymphoma, CLL, melanoma, or a variety of solid tumors took the medication as outpatients. The most prevalent toxicities were fatigue (71 percent), nausea (69 percent), hypotension (51 percent), and weight gain (37 percent). Four participants died of unrelated causes during the first 2 weeks of therapy. Twenty-three patients stopped treatment before completing the course because of progressive disease (12), severe hypotension (3), azotemia (1), myocardial infarction (1), early death (4), and miscellaneous causes (2). Four of 12 patients with malignant lymphoma or CLL responded, 3 partially and 1 with a minor response, lasting 1 to 17[+] months. The authors concluded that a dose of 1 mg was moderately toxic but that a dose of 0.5 mg was tolerable for out-patients.[73]

Substantial antitumor effects have been seen only with quite high doses of IL-2, levels approaching the range at which toxicity occurs.[74] IL-2 seems to promote an associated release of other lymphokines, such as gamma-interferon and tumor-necrosis factor, that can damage endothelium and lead to a "capillary-leak syndrome" and massive fluid retention;[5] gamma-interferon has been demonstrated in the circulation after treatment with IL-2.[66,75] This problem illustrates the enigma constantly encountered with the use of immunomodulators and other biologic response modifiers—the body's system of interconnections and interrelations is so complicated, intricate, and all-embracing that, when one member is disturbed or altered, repercussions are very apparent from other members.

The early reports of LAK cells[76,77] prompted doubts regarding the differentiation between LAK and NK cells. Many researchers believe that results attributed to LAK cells may have been due to increased NK cell activity. Lotzová and Herberman wrote that

> the general consensus of the leading laboratories in the field is the following: (1) LAK is not a unique cell type but a phenomenon, a function of cells; (2) most of the peripheral blood, splenic and bone marrow LAK activity is mediated by IL-2-activated NK cells; (3) in most instances, no or very low LAK activity is generated from cultures depleted of NK cells; (4) T cells have also been described to contribute to the LAK phenomenon, but their contribution in peripheral blood, bone marrow and spleen appears to be minor.[78]

The creation of recombinant IL-2 has stimulated research in the use of this lymphokine as a therapeutic agent.

COLONY-STIMULATING FACTORS (CSFs)

As early as 1884, Metschnikoff[79] raised the possibility of using phagocytes against organisms that cause disease,[80] and by 1903

Wright and Douglas[81] had investigated the role of blood fluids in phagocytosis.[80] Therefore, the very recent theories of stimulating the production of leukocytes in the cancer battle have historic precedent.

In 1906, Carnot and Deflandre[82] showed that "a humoral factor, termed erythropoietin, was involved in the regulation of erythropoiesis."[83] The next milestone was reached in 1961 with the report by Till and McCulloch[84] that, when viable bone marrow cells are injected into lethally irradiated mice, distinct nodules appear in the spleen of the recipient.[85] Becker, McCulloch, and Till (1963) found that each such nodule is the progeny of one cell, designated as a colony-forming unit, and, hence, that colonies are clones.[86]

Two years later (1965), Pluznik and Sachs cloned normal mouse "mast" cells in tissue culture in a soft agar medium and showed that colony formation required the presence of an embryo-cell feeder layer.[87] Wing and Shadduck reported that, "surprisingly, the colonies formed in these cultures consisted of only granulocytes and macrophages."[88]

The discovery of colony-stimulating factor occurred promptly after colonies of hematopoietic cells were successfully grown in vitro.[88] Virtually all colonies "are initially composed of granulocytic cells but on continued incubation macrophages appear in most aggregates and eventually comprise the sole population."[89]

The stem cell is a generalized mother cell that can proliferate and differentiate along several pathways, resulting in the various blood elements.[88,90] Yoffey described the hematopoietic stem cell as "a cell which does not possess any of the signs of differentiation in its cytoplasm or nucleus but is nevertheless capable of differentiating into an erythrocyte, granulocyte, monocyte or megakaryocyte."[91]

In 1968, Wolf and Trentin wrote that their research supported "the working hypothesis derived from earlier spleen colony studies regarding the influence of the organ micro-environment on the line of hemopoietic differentiation within a colony. In the bone marrow cavity ... most early colonies were found to be granuloid, whereas in the spleen ... most early colonies were erythroid."[85] Thus, "the stroma of tissues containing stem cells influences the type of differentiation and the degree of proliferation that occurs."[88]

Subsequently, investigators have shown that factors necessary for hematopoietic cell multiplication are specific for each cell line and even for each period of cell differentiation.[88] For example, Stephenson et al. (1971) established that erythropoietin is necessary for erythroid colonies to form. As they summarized: "A method has been presented for obtaining colonies of erythroid cells in cultures of hemopoietic cells from the liver of 13-day mouse fetuses. The development of these colonies was shown to depend on the presence of the hormone erythropoietin in the medium, and the colonies were shown to be composed of hemoglobin-synthesizing cells."[92] The factors that actuate eosinophil and megakaryocyte colonies have also been characterized.[88]

T cells furnish the first two of the four known CSFs (IL-3, granulocyte-macrophage [GM]-CSF, granulocyte [G]-CSF, and macrophage [M]-CSF), that regulate multiplication and differentiation of granulocytes and macrophages.[93] (IL-3 has also been labeled multicolony CSF.) The CSFs are named from the cell lineage they stimulate. Thus, granulocyte colonies are stimulated by G-CSF, macrophage colonies by M-CSF, and mixed colonies of granulocytes and macrophages by GM-CSF. The administration of G-CSF, however, causes prominent increases in neutrophils only and not in other granular leukocytes; GM-CSF increases the number of neutrophils, eosinophils, and monocytes.[94] Also, some authors have used different terminology for the CSFs, such as alpha, beta or CSF-1, 2, etc.[95]

A relatively pure preparation of GM-CSF was obtained from human urine, and the molecule was shown to be a glycoprotein with an apparent molecular weight of 45,000 (1969).[83,96] In 1975, the gene for human GM-CSF was found to reside on the long arm of chromosome 5,[97] and this gene was cloned (1985) by Cantrell et al.[98] and also by Wong and colleagues.[99]

Under normal conditions, the immature cells in the bone marrow grow and differentiate into the mature cells usually seen in the peripheral blood. In most leukemias, there is an excess of immature cells in both the bone marrow and the circulating blood. These leukemia cells have come to a standstill or halted at an early period of differentiation. However, they retain the ability to duplicate themselves. At present, we do not know whether this disturbance in maturation could sometimes be due to a deficiency of a maturation factor. As Chiao and Lutton stated:

> With the accumulation of evidence that various leukemia cells can be induced to differentiate, scientists have attempted to understand the mechanism underlying the process of differentiation induction and to characterize the inducer molecules. Since some types of leukemia cells are frozen at specific differentiation stages of the hematopoietic process, the induction of terminal differentiation by certain inducers may be a viable approach to the therapy of the leukemias.[95]

At present, most of the information regarding the use of growth or differentiating factors against cancer is the result of in vitro or animal research. Moore wrote: "Despite such limitations, the data nevertheless present a strong argument that the apparent block in maturation associated with neoplastic transformation is a reversible event, that transformed cells retain some dependence on regulatory factors of endogenous or exogenous origin, and that manipulation of such factors has a role in cancer therapy."[100]

Moore believes that the first explicit data showing that cells can be influenced to change from a malignant to a normal phenotype were those presented in 1971 by Friend et al.[101] They reported "on a virally induced erythroleukemia in mice that responded to treatment with dimethylsulfoxide (DMSO) by differentiating, as shown by hemoglobin synthesis in formerly hemoglobin-negative leukemic cell lines."[100] Their conclusion was that "perhaps an interference in the normal flow of information from DNA into cell proteins results in malignancy. It may now be possible to ascertain if agents such as DMSO influence part(s) of the genome of the malignant cell to permit it to mature fully to the stage of its normal counterpart."[101]

Since that article, many substances with the capability of influencing differentiation have been identified. Synthetic retinoids (vitamin A analogs) can stimulate myeloid leukemic cells, notably the HL-60 line, to differentiate in vitro.[100] Abe et al. (1981) suggested "the possibility that the active form of vitamin D_3 is involved in the differentiation of bone marrow cells. . . . [It] was capable of inducing differentiation of myeloid leukemia cells into macrophages."[102]

Only a few human studies using GM-CSF have been reported. Gerhartz and Wilmanns (1986) tested the prognostic value of in vitro cloning of bone marrow and blood cells from 32 patients with acute myeloid leukemia. Poor response to GM-CSF in vitro seemed to be associated with poor survival. This could not be proven statistically, probably because of the small number of cases. Serial bone marrow cultures during the first complete remission showed that, over time, the number of colony-forming cells gradually declined. Peripheral-blood colony-forming cells, however, proved to be a more valuable predictive test for imminent relapse. A patient with low colony numbers in the peripheral blood is at a high risk of early relapse.[103]

According to Vadhan-Raj et al. (1987), "The myelodysplastic syndromes are a group of stem-cell disorders characterized by maturation defects resulting in ineffective hematopoiesis, refractory cytopenias often leading to infection or hemorrhage, and an increased risk of leukemic transformation."[104] They go on to state that there is no consistently effective treatment, although retinoids, vitamin D analogs, and cytotoxic drugs have been tried. They used recombinant human GM-CSF to treat eight patients who had myelodysplasias. The factor was given by continuous i.v. infusion daily for 2 weeks, and then this regimen was repeated after a 2-week rest. All eight patients showed marked increases in peripheral blood leukocytes (5- to 70-fold), including granulocytes (5- to 373-fold). The absolute numbers of monocytes, eosinophils, and lymphocytes increased in all patients. Three of the eight also had increases in platelet counts and improvement in erythropoiesis to the extent that two persons who had required platelet and red cell transfusions no longer needed them. Side effects were mild to moderate bone pain, fever, chills, myalgias, headache, decreased appetite, and nausea.[104]

The following year (1988), Vadhan-Raj and associates gave GM-CSF to 10 patients who had moderate or severe aplastic anemia. They used a similar treatment schedule. The white cell count increased in all patients primarily because of an increase in the numbers of neutrophils, eosinophils, and monocytes. Side effects were mild to moderate and included bone pain, gastrointestinal disturbances, itching, and occasional swelling of wrists and ankles.[105] It seems that GM-CSF has relatively low toxicity when compared with IL-2 and tumor-necrosis factor.[106]

According to Cosman, Mertelsmann (University of Mainz) related that blast cell levels increased in some patients with myelodysplasia after the administration of GM-CSF. These persons had >20% blasts in the marrow before therapy, suggesting that care must be taken in selecting patients for GM-CSF therapy.[106]

As Groopman (1988) wrote: "Another concern regarding GM-CSF therapy for patients with myelodysplasia is whether the development of acute leukemia may be accelerated. . . . Presumably, leukemic cells of myeloid origin have receptors for GM-CSF, and so GM-CSF may expand this population. This uneasiness is supported by reports that leukemia blasts have been stimulated by GM-CSF in a few patients."[107]

"It is not known whether antibodies to GM-CSF may develop that can abrogate the hematologic response."[107] Therapy with GM-CSF may create a "potential for increase in the incidence or severity of graft-vs-host disease following allogeneic bone marrow transplantation."[94]

On the positive side, Gabrilove cited three areas:

The growth factors may . . . prove useful in augmenting the number of malignant cells recruited into the S phase of the cell cycle, thereby enhancing the susceptibility of these cells to killing by cycle-specific agents such as cytosine arabinoside.

Both G-CSF and GM-CSF have been shown to increase peripheral blood hematopoietic progenitors.[108] This should allow peripheral blood to be used as a vehicle for autologous or possibly allogeneic transplantation, perhaps obviating the need for bone marrow harvesting.

Finally, CSFs—G-CSF and M-CSF in particular—may be useful in diminishing leukemic cell self-renewal by promoting cell maturation. By promoting terminal cell maturation, one might be able to extinguish the leukemic clone.[109]

The biologic response modifiers represent a very active and vigorous area of cancer research at present, and the past decade has witnessed a great surge of information about them. Interferons are of proven value against hairy cell leukemia, CML, and T cell lymphomas, but the potential worth of other BRMs remains to be determined. Animal studies have shown that some of these biologic response modifiers offer powerful prophylaxis against the development of cancer, and BRMs may, eventually, prove to be useful in cancer prevention.[110] Also, there is evidence that BRMs that stimulate NK cell activity offer substantial protection against the spread of malignant tumors; this approach to preventing the metastatic dissemination of tumor cells is under investigation.[110]

EIGHT

Human Cytogenetics

Genes are independent sorts
Assorting independently
Which intertwine and recombine
Much more than incidentally.

CANDACE GALEN, "Diversity's the Splice of Life"

CYTOLOGIC BACKGROUND

Researchers viewed human chromosomes for the first time in the 1870s when suitable staining and fixation techniques became available. The word *chromosome* was devised and first used by Wilhelm Waldeyer in an 1888 publication,[1] which was translated into English in 1889.[2]

In the first place I must beg leave to propose a separate technical name "chromosome" for those things which have been called by Boveri "chromatic elements," in which there occurs one of the most important acts in karyokinesis, viz. the longitudinal splitting. . . . "Chromatic elements" is too long. On the other hand they are so important that a special and shorter name appears useful. . . . If the one I propose is practically applicable it will become familiar, otherwise it will soon sink into oblivion.[2,3]

Because the early cytologists saw chromosomes as bodies that stained with colored dyes, Waldeyer combined the Greek *chroma* for color and *soma* for body.[4]

As techniques in staining and microscopy improved, Arnold (1879)[5] was able to describe chromosomes of human malignant tumor cells.[3] The initial publication depicting the normal chromosomes in humans, however, seems to be that of Flemming in 1882,[6] in which he included drawings of the "various phases of cellular division in human normal cells."[7] Working later with human cornea cells, Flemming (1889)[8] reported that the normal number of chromosomes in humans ranged from 22 to 24.[7] Not only was Flemming an expert cytologist, he also formulated a fixative solution that, according to Baker, was still unsurpassed for chromosome study as recently as 1950. It consisted of osmic acid (osmium tetroxide), chromic acid, and acetic acid and was so successful because the damage caused by one ingredient (such as shrinking due to chromic acid) was counteracted by the damage from another (such as swelling due to acetic acid).[9,10]

By the late 1880s, the concept that hereditary traits were transmitted by chromosomes aroused two schools of thought. Some argued that the number of chromosomes in cells was unchangeable because chromosomes were enduring and permanent; other scientists believed that chromosomes were temporary structures that could separate into granules in the resting cell nucleus and reorganize with each cell division.[9]

This controversy provoked interest in chromosome numbers, and cytologists began attempts to count them. Results for humans differed extensively from 8 to over 50, but the predominant counts were around 24 in diploid cells and 12 in haploid cells. These numbers remained in many textbooks as late as 1930.[9] Kottler explained why low chromosome counts were the norm for all mammalian species examined during that period: cytologists generally used tissues from corpses, and chromosomes in dead cells clump together very rapidly.[9]

Winiwarter

Winiwarter was the first to realize that, to count chromosomes, fresh tissue is imperative, and it must be fixed immediately on removal from the body. He was also the first to maintain that chromosomes formed side-by-side pairs during the synapsis stage of the first maturation division.[9,11] Winiwarter's meticulous labors produced chromosome preparations that far surpassed those of others of his day. For human studies, he used fresh testis removed surgically and fixed immediately with Flemming's mixture.[9]

In 1912, Winiwarter published studies on human spermatogenesis, counting 47 chromosomes in spermatogonia and 48 in oogonia.[12] His findings contradicted the accepted doctrine that human cells contained only 24 chromosomes. According to Kottler:

> [Winiwarter found that] primary spermatocytes possessed 24 chromosomes, one of which appeared and behaved differently from the other 23. During the first maturation division Winiwarter saw this unusual chromosome pass undivided to only one of the two poles. Thus, in the two anaphase groups formed during a primary spermatocyte division, Winiwarter counted 24 chromosomes in one but just 23 in the other. Accordingly, secondary spermatocytes were of two varieties, with 23 or 24 chromosomes. Winiwarter concluded that males were of the XO sex chromosome type, known for over a decade in insects. In spermatogonia, there were 46 autosomes and one X sex chromosome. In primary spermatocytes, there were 23 bivalents and one X. Among secondary spermatocytes, some possessed 23 autosomes and one X, while others possessed just 23 autosomes. If the male were of the XO type, the female should be of the XX type, with a total of 48 chromosomes.[9]

Although Winiwarter's counts were not disproved, the accepted teaching was still that human cells contained 24 chromosomes.

Painter

Then, in the 1920s, Painter (who later became president of the University of Texas) began working on human chromosomes. He had been interested in genetics since his college days at Yale; his thesis was on spider spermatogenesis. Around 1920, he published a comprehensive account of spermatogenesis in reptiles and then embarked on a study of mammalian chromosomes because there was a profusion of available material. "There was 'possum meat all over the lab,"[9] as Kottler tells us, because a colleague was working on opossum reproduction.

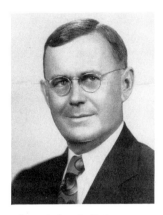

Theophilus S. Painter

The sex chromosomes in the opossum are very small and easily recognizable. It was no problem for Painter to count the chromosomes (22) and identify the X and Y sex chromosomes in spermatogonia and primary spermatocytes. He found the two X chromosomes that he had expected in the female somatic cells. His positive identification of these X and Y chromosomes gave him an advantage in his subsequent work with the more complex delineation in humans.[9] Referring to his first work with human chromosomes, Painter later said that he "happened to be in the right place at the right time, for one of [his] former premedical students was practicing in a state mental institution in Austin where, for therapeutic reasons (excessive self abuse coupled with certain phases of insanity which made the removal of the sex glands desirable), they occasionally castrated male individuals."[9] The testes removed from three inmates (one white and two black) were minced and immediately fixed. In May 1921, Painter wrote that spermatogonia from both races contained between 45 and 48 chromosomes.[13] In primary spermatocytes, Painter found two chromosomes that looked and behaved just like the X and Y opossum chromosomes. Therefore, he concluded that humans were of the XY/XX sex chromosome type and hence should have an even number of diploid chromosomes, either 46 or 48. As he stated: "In the clearest equatorial plates so far studied only 46 chromosomes have been found. Before a final conclusion is made on the exact number it is desired to make a careful study of a large number of division plates."[13] By September 1921, however, Painter had decided in favor of 48 chromosomes.[9,14,15] He remained firmly convinced that his work had established unequivocally the presence of both X and Y chromosomes in spermatogonia.[9]

Although Winiwarter disagreed with Painter and adhered to his original belief, Painter's conclusions were confirmed by experts all over the world. For the next 35 years there was no longer any controversy—human cells contained 48 chromosomes. As late as 1954, cytologist Leo Sachs declared, "The existence of an XY sex mechanism and of the diploid chromosome number of 48 in man can therefore now be considered as an established fact."[16]

Tjio and Levan

Just 1 year later (in December 1955) Tjio and Levan counted just 46 chromosomes in human embryonic lung cells. This was a startling and totally unanticipated finding for them. After corroboration by 260 repeat counts, they published their findings in 1956.[17] Rightfully, they are given credit for the landmark report of the corrected chromosome number in humans.

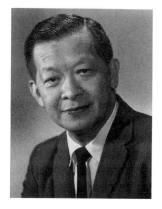

Tjio and Levan were able to make accurate counts repeatedly and quickly because of improvements in cytologic techniques. Hsu wrote a very interesting historic account of these developments from his personal viewpoint as one of the prominent participants.[18] Before the 1920s, chro-

Joe Hin Tjio

mosome studies were performed on traditional paraffin sections; in preparing these sections, the technician often sliced cells and even long chromosomes into several segments, causing confusion and errors in counting. In 1921, Belling introduced a better process, the squash technique. "When the preparation is a day or two old, the cytoplasm has swollen; and a slight tap on the thin coverglass above any particular cell will usually free the cytoplasm from the cell wall, and another tap flatten it out with its contained chromosomes."[19] Squashing preserved the cell and the chromosomes intact and was of additional benefit because flattening the cell frequently separated the chromosomes and placed them all in one plane of focus.[18]

Adding colchicine before fixing the specimens was the next substantial advance in cytologic technique. This alkaloid interrupts the organization of the mitotic spindle and halts cell division at metaphase (Blakeslee and Avery, 1937;[20] Levan, 1938[21]). Thus, colchicine treatment increases the number of mitotic cells available for observing chromosomes.[18] It also contracts the chromosomes, decreasing the probability of chromosome overlap.[9]

In the early 1950s, tissue culture (cells grown outside the body in a nutrient medium) came into common use. These cells were treated with colchicine several hours before fixation and with a hypotonic salt solution several minutes before fixation.[9] A hypotonic solution disperses metaphase chromosomes, an occurrence that had been noted by several researchers at least as early as 1934.[22] The information had not been disseminated, and in 1952 three reports mentioned its rediscovery.[23–25] Hsu described his accidental recognition of this phenomenon when he used a salt solution that a laboratory worker had erroneously made hypotonic. He couldn't believe his eyes when he saw beautifully scattered mitotic chromosomes with no spindle orientation.[18] The experience led him to comment, "It only shows that to achieve some discovery, sloppy technicians are occasionally helpful."[26] Hsu (1952) was probably the first to use both colchicine and hypotonic solution to pretreat cells for human chromosome study.[25] Cells grown in tissue culture are unusually large, and the hypotonic pretreatment swells them further and dissolves the spindle.[9]

This improved cytologic technique was used by Tjio and Levan (1956) and aided them in obtaining good metaphase spreads, from which they could make an accurate revision of the chromosome number.[9] Many authors agree with Court-Brown that "modern human cytogenetics dates from 1956 when it was established that the human diploid chromosome number was 46. This discovery and the technical advances making it possible opened the way for the investigation of abnormal states of development that might be linked to an abnormal chromosome constitution."[27]

EARLY MEDICAL CYTOGENETICS

As mentioned in chapter 2, Boveri (1902) advanced the supposition that malignant tumors could be the result of an abnormal chromosome composition.[28] The Boveri hypothesis (1914)[29] includes the concepts that a malignant tumor cell has an abnormal chromosome composition and that any circumstance that causes such a deviation results in a malignancy.[3] He believed that malignant cells developed from normal cells and that the source of the deviant behavior lay solely in the tumor cell, not in the environment.[30] Boveri also introduced the theory of the monoclonal origin of cancer, writing, "typically each tumor takes its origin from one and a single cell."[3,29] Boveri would probably be astonished if he could know that 75 years later "the problems and questions related to the role of chromosomal changes in the genesis of neoplasia would still occasion deep controversy."[3]

Conjectures that some congenital aberrations might be caused by chromosomal irregularities were recorded in the 1930s. Waardenburg (1932)[31] urged "cytologists to consider the possibility that in mongolism lies an example of specific chromosome aberration in man . . . perhaps a chromosome deficiency through nondisjunction or the reverse, a chromosome duplication."[18]

Lejeune

After the Tjio and Levan report appeared, Lejeune began examining chromosomes of children with Down's syndrome. In the specimen from a 2-year-old boy, he distinctly counted 47, trisomic for one of the smallest chromosomes (now known as number 21),

Metaphase from a human embryonic lung cell culture as seen by Tjio on December 22, 1955, at 2:00 A.M.

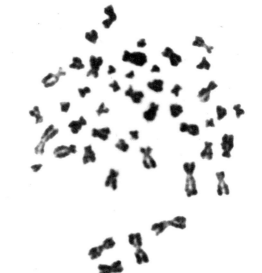

and was amazed when he subsequently found the same peculiarity in a second and a third patient. He presented his findings at a seminar in 1958, and the publication by Lejeune and colleagues appeared in 1959.[32] This was the first description of a chromosomal abnormality associated with a human disease. Hsu provided an unforgettable description of the laboratory facilities in which Lejeune accomplished this momentous research: He had no running water, but there was a faucet in a tiny kitchen-like room next door; he borrowed a discarded microscope with gears so worn that the arm could not be adjusted, and he used a piece of tinfoil from a candy wrapper to stabilize the mechanism; he had no photographic equipment and arranged to use some belonging to the pathology department for 2 hours each week; he required the apparatus and proficiency necessary to establish cell cultures, and a colleague's laboratory assistant knew the techniques and was willing to help. His historic project, from start to publication, cost about $200.[18]

Dissemination of the article by Lejeune et al. brought worldwide confirmation of their findings and verification of the conclusion that all patients with Down's syndrome exhibit the same trisomy. Other congenital disorders were soon investigated, and cytogeneticists determined that human chromosomes are not fixed or constant; conversely, deviations from what is considered normal show up commonly and with no apparent provocation.

Denver Classification

By 1960, teams of scientists from many countries were analyzing the human karyotype. A karyotype is a photomicrograph of chromosomes arranged into groups according to size and similarities. Many researchers devised their own schemes of terminology, which led to confusion in interpreting published reports. Because Ford of the Medical Research Council in England stressed that a standard system of nomenclature should be instituted, Puck made arrangements for a conference to be held in Denver in April 1960.[18] He chose three moderators, Catcheside (Birmingham), Muller (Bloomington), and Stern (Berkeley). The participants were all prominent investigators in that sphere of research: Böök (Uppsala), Chu (Oak Ridge), Ford (Harwell), Fraccaro (Uppsala), Harnden (Edinburgh), Hsu (Houston), Hungerford (Philadelphia), Jacobs

(Edinburgh), Lejeune (Paris), Levan (Lund), Makino (Sapporo), Puck (Denver), Robinson (Denver), and Tjio (Bethesda).[18] Over 4 days, they worked out a mutually acceptable plan of grouping chromosomes according to size and numbering each pair from 1 to 22; they called the sex chromosomes X and Y. Pätau (1961) proposed using letters (alphabetically A through G) to designate the groups. Although many pairs within a chromosome group could not be identified positively at that time (this came later when banding techniques were developed),[18] use of the Denver classification brought order to the literature. Subsequent conferences in London (1963), Chicago (1966), Paris (1971), Stockholm (1977), Jerusalem (1981), and Berlin (1985) resulted in updated recommendations.

BANDING

Q-banding

The technique of banding, which was introduced in the late 1960s and early 1970s, proved to be a major advance for identifying and differentiating chromosomes. Hsu explained that, in the late 1960s, Caspersson, of the Karolinska Institute in Stockholm, was a consultant to the Children's Cancer Research Foundation in Boston. Caspersson was an authority in fluorometry and suggested attaching an alkylating agent to a fluorochrome molecule to determine whether the agent might "crosslink guanines of the DNA in the chromosomes [so that] the stain would give fluorescence. Then if the distribution of base pairs along a chromosome is nonrandom, the guanine-cytosine-rich areas should receive more crosslinking of this compound molecule than adenine-thymine-rich areas, consequently showing brighter fluorescence."[18] He suspected that a chromosome might have zones of bright and dim fluorescence. An organic chemist in Boston synthesized such a compound (quinacrine mustard), and it was shipped to Stockholm for testing. Caspersson and colleagues reported their first studies with plant chromosomes in 1969[33] and, 1 year later, published findings on human chromosomes.[34] Pairs could be recognized by their patterns of fluorescent banding. Later, it was shown that the degree of brightness correlates with the base composition—those with high adenine thymine (AT) ratios give brighter fluorescence than those with low AT ratios.[18] At the Paris Conference in 1971, it was decided to label this phenomenon *quinacrine* or *Q-banding*.[18]

G-banding

Gustav Giemsa (1867–1948) was a chemist and bacteriologist in Hamburg who developed a stain designed to identify protozoan parasites in blood preparations. As Hsu wrote:

> The popularity of Giemsa stain among human and mammalian cytogeneticists probably stemmed from Peter Nowell. When Peter was studying human lymphocyte cultures, he naturally used the Giemsa blood stain. When Paul Moorhead and his associates (including Nowell) described their lymphocyte culture method for human cytogenetic preparations, their recipe called for Giemsa staining. This procedure has been so reproducible and so convenient that practically all human cytogeneticists (and, later, mammalian cytogeneticists) followed.[18]

Chromosome preparations with Giemsa stain at pH 9.0 show deeply stained bands that are characteristic for each chromosome. In 1971, three papers outlining techniques for Giemsa (G) banding were published.[35–37]

C-banding

Constitutive heterochromatin banding was discovered in 1970 by Arrighi and Hsu, who then submitted a manuscript to *Lancet.*

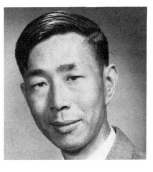

The editor returned the paper, stating that the article had no medical application; it was then published the following year in *Cytogenetics.*[38] Also in 1971, other scientists reported heterochromatin staining procedures.[39,40] It has been determined that whenever highly repetitive DNA sequences are present a C-band shows up, regardless of base composition.[18] The function of these sequences is not understood, and they are frequently referred to as

Tao-Chiuh Hsu

junk DNA. Dark C-bands are found at the centromeres (constricted portions) of all chromosomes except the Y, which instead stains heavily on the distal region of the long arm.[41] C-bands vary markedly, and, in the human population, practically no two individuals have identical heterochromatin patterns.[18] C-banding is used to explore chromosome rearrangement near centromeres and to investigate polymorphism.[41]

R-banding

Reverse banding was discovered by Dutrillaux and Lejeune (1971)[42] when they heated cytologic preparations in hot phosphate buffer and then stained them with Giemsa. The bands are the opposite of the G-bands, i.e., dark G-bands appear pale with the R technique while light G-bands stain darkly. R-banding is of value in determining chromosome ends. In humans, the terminal regions of most chromosomes are light with G-banding and dim with Q-banding, but they stand out brilliantly with R-banding.[18]

Trypsin Technique

Two separate articles, published within 2 months, introduced the trypsin treatment for quick slide preparation (Seabright, November 1971;[43] Wang and Fedoroff, January 1972[44]); trypsin hydrolyzes the protein component of nucleoprotein. This technique was soon adopted by cytologists because it produced an improved chromosome display that was ready for viewing about 10 minutes after starting with air-dried material.[43] Wang and Fedoroff undertook their experiments to ascertain whether "removal of the protein component of the nucleoprotein complexes making up the chromosomes might then allow Giemsa stain to react directly with the nucleic acid component."[44]

Numerous other staining methods and combinations of stains have been described, and many are in use today. Some clarify specific areas of chromosomes and are employed when the need arises. However, for routine procedures, Giemsa-banding with various modifications of the trypsin technique have been most widely used. Today, with techniques called "high resolution," chromosome bands are being further segmented into subbands, etc., for even more precise analyses.[45] With these methods, abnormalities are being recorded in a very high percentage of patients with certain leukemias.

KARYOTYPIC PATTERNS IN LEUKEMIAS

Chromosomes are classified according to standardized terminology that was defined at the Paris Conference (1971) and amended in succeeding years. Briefly, the long arm is designated *q*, the short arm *p*, a loss or gain of a whole chromosome is expressed by − or +, respectively, before the chromosome number, and either of those symbols after a chromosome indicates a loss or gain of part of the chromosome. Translocation (*t*) is the shifting of a fragment between chromosomes, with the affected chromosomes in parentheses and the breakpoints also indicated. For example, t(8;21)(q22;q22) translates into an exchange between chromosomes 8 and 21; the breakpoint in each chromosome is on the long arm, region 2, band 2. The fragments distal to the breakpoints have traded places. Deletion (*del*) indicates that a part of the chromosome has been lost, and inversion (*inv*) signifies that a chromosome has broken at two points and reunited with the middle segment inverted. For example, if sections along a chromosome are labeled *a, b, c, d*, an inversion would produce *a, c, b, d*. With high resolution precision, the subband number follows a punctuation period after the band number. Therefore, 8q22.2 pinpoints chromosome 8, the long arm, region 2, band 2, subband 2.

To ascertain karyotypic changes in patients with cancer, the malignant cells must be analyzed; all cells in each cancer are progeny of a single source cell, and they all exhibit the genetic peculiarities that exist in the original cancer cell. Body tissues that are uninvolved with the cancer have normal chromosome constitutions. Frequently, however, cancer tissue is not attainable or does not exhibit a sufficient number of metaphases. Although certain mitogenic substances stimulate T and B cells to divide, many other cell types, especially those of malignant origin, cannot, as yet, be provoked into active mitosis.[46] Sandberg commented, "Often chromosomes of cancers are contracted and changes are complex and numerous, so detailed analysis is impossible even with the best banding techniques."[46] The majority of human cancers have not been explored thoroughly because the cytologic pictures are so complex as almost to defy analysis.[18]

During the 1970s, examinations of cancer cells showed that most had karyologic aberrations, but there did not seem to be consistent patterns of irregularity in cancers of the same cell type. Hsu (1979) stated, "In fact, even in the same animal or in the same patient, the chromosome composition may change considerably as the tumor progresses."[18] As a result, researchers have been reluctant to relate chromosomal changes to the etiology of cancer.

Since Nowell and Hungerford (1960) first recognized a chromosome abnormality in two patients with CML, leukemia study has been in the forefront of research concerning the diagnostic relevance of chromosome aberrations. Before staining techniques were available, cytogenetic abnormalities were known to exist in about 40 to 60 percent of patients with acute leukemia, but these abnormalities were considered to be random and not specific to any type of acute leukemia. This situation was different from that of CGL, in which a high percentage of patients had the characteristic Ph^1 chromosome. When researchers attained experience and competence with the new staining procedures, however, they learned that certain karyotypic abnormalities were nonrandom and had diagnostic and prognostic implications. Rowley (1989) wrote that, by 1976, it had become clear that particular chromosome changes were associated with specific types of leukemia; her group could identify certain changes that were uniquely and, in some instances, invariably associated with a specific type of acute leukemia.[47]

Sandberg (1977) may have been the first to report using cytogenetic data to influence the selection of therapy.[48] He determined that treatment actually reduced the life span of a patient with leukemia if all of the cells in the bone marrow had cytogenetic deviations. If normal cells were interspersed, however, therapy was likely to be beneficial by reducing the number of abnormal cells.[49]

Scientists from many countries have been engaged in cancer cytogenetic research, and they have repeatedly encountered evidence showing that chromosomal divergence is nonrandom. In one of the earliest reported studies, Manolov and Manolova (1972) found an extra terminal band on a number 14 chromosome from 10 of 12 patients with Burkitt lymphoma.[18,50] Four years later, Zech et al. substantiated that alteration and reported that the terminal band was missing from a number 8 chromosome.[51] Apparently a categoric translocation is the modification in that cancer.[18] Dofuku and colleagues (1975)[52] found that a chromosome 15 trisomy was the abnormality in the leukemias of the AKR strain of mice.[18]

Although nonrandom changes occur in chromosomes of human leukemia and other cancers, Sandberg (1980) believes that "they are a reflection of events tangential to the basic causation of these diseases, with a small number of nonrandom chromosomal lesions reflecting a susceptibility of some chromosomes or their regions to the influences of the already existing neoplastic condition."[3]

By the 1980s, extensive data on chromosomal changes and neoplasia had been collected. Probably the most thorough investigations of the relationships between cytogenetic aberrations, prognosis, and therapy were conducted by Mitelman.[53,54] He assembled the current knowledge on chromosomal abnormalities in leukemia and related it to duration of remissions and treatment.[49] Sandberg also extensively described chromosomes in cancers, including leukemia (1980).[3] In spite of diligent efforts to catalog them, the vast array of data and the very complex nature of the changes make for much confusion. Cruciger and associates (1976), in an attempt to solve this problem, analyzed seven human breast carcinomas, each having complex chromosomal abnormalities.[55] Instead of characterizing every change, they determined whether one or more changes were shared by all tumors. They discovered one common denominator, a marker chromosome always involving the long arm of chromosome number 1. In all cases, 1q was involved in a translocation, but the recipient chromosomes differed.[18]

This same principle has been pursued by other cytogeneticists, who have searched for chromosomal abnormalities shared by tumor specimens of the same pathologic type. They have realized that tumors classified as a single type by pathologists may actually represent several different genetic origins. For example, cases of CML that do not manifest the Ph[1] chromosome may have a genetic origin different from those that do. The practice of using hematologic criteria for diagnosis caused them to be lumped together as one disorder.[18] Sandberg (1980) stated that eventually the label CML may have to be limited to those patients exhibiting the Ph[1] chromosome.[3] Subsequent studies (as described in chapter 2) showed that the diagnosis of CML may have to be confined to those patients having the *bcr-abl* rearrangement, whether they are Ph positive or negative.

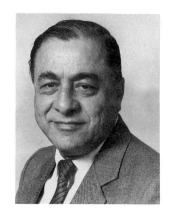

José M. Trujillo

Over the past 15 years, extensive evidence has related cytogenetic abnormalities to the clinical course of patients with acute leukemia. The suspicion of such a correlation was reported in 1974 by Trujillo et al. They determined median survival times for adults with diploid and aneuploid acute leukemia and also compared survival curves of patients with diploid karyotypes to those of persons in the three main categories of aneuploidy (hypodiploid, pseudodiploid, and hyperdiploid). They concluded that analysis of survival times "suggested that some of these abnormal cytogenetic profiles may have definite clinical implications."[56]

ANLL

At the Fourth International Workshop on Chromosomes in Leukemia (1982), laboratory statistics for patients investigated showed that 53.7 percent of patients with de novo ANLL and 75 percent of patients with ANLL secondary to cytotoxic therapy had abnormal karyotypic patterns.[57] Yunis et al. reported that all patients with ANLL may have a chromosomal defect.[58]

According to Rowley, "The first consistent translocation in ANLL was detected in patients with AML; it occurs in about 15% of aneuploid patients with AML . . . and involves the long arms of Nos. 8 and 21, t(8q−;21q+)."[59] Using quinacrine fluorescence, Rowley discovered this translocation and reported it in 1973.[60] It is frequently accompanied by the loss of a sex chromosome, and the cells of affected persons tend to contain Auer rods.[59]

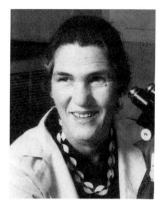

Janet D. Rowley

Trujillo et al. (1979) described 32 patients with acute granulocytic leukemia, all of whom presented a specific type of aneuploidy identified as a translocation of numbers 8 and 21.[61] The authors had previously (1974) reported and categorized these consistent karyotypic changes as the "complex" profile.[56] Among the 32 patients studied, the Y chromosome was missing in 8 of 19 men, and 1 of the 2 X chromosomes was absent in 2 of 13 women. The cells of all patients contained Auer rods.

Adults showing this alteration have a greater than 90 percent probability of achieving complete remission and they seem to have a good prospect for prolonged survival.[62] It is the single most common structural reorganization in patients with ANLL.

Arthur and Bloomfield (1983) described patients with ANLL whose bone marrow eosinophils were significantly increased. All had a partial deletion of the long arm of number 16, del(16)(q22).[63] That same year, LeBeau and associates reported finding inv(16)(p13q22);[64] practically all patients with this inversion had abnormal eosinophils, although only about two thirds showed an increase in the number of eosinophils.[65] Over 90 percent of the patients showing inv(16) achieve complete remission with Ara-C and an anthracycline combination, and, in general, the group enjoys a favorable prognosis. Among those who do develop recurrent disease, however, a high percentage suffer central nervous system relapse with intracerebral leukemic nodules. About 7 percent of the patients with AML show the inv(16) cytologic pattern.[62,66]

Golomb et al. (1976) described a partial deletion of the long arm of chromosome 17 in two patients with acute promyelocytic leukemia;[67] this was later characterized as a translocation between chromosomes 15 and 17.[68] Golomb's group at the University of Chicago subsequently (1984) described the translocation in each of 27 patients with acute promyelocytic leukemia from whom satisfactory cytogenetic specimens were available.[69] The translocation seems to be diagnostic for that particular leukemia and has not been found in patients from any other subgroup.[70] Patients exhibiting t(15;17), however, have an extraordinarily high incidence of hemorrhagic diathesis associated with the disease and often aggravated early in the treatment regimen. This occurrence constitutes a medical emergency and requires aggressive administration of procoagulants and platelets. Although the risk of death during induction is high, for the patients who achieve complete remission the prospect for long-term survival is excellent.[66]

In patients with ANLL, the most common deviations that affect whole chromosomes are a gain of one number 8 or a loss of one number 7, and often either of these is the only irregularity in leukemic cells. Apparently these changes are not associated with a specific subtype of leukemia.[59] Philip and colleagues (1977) described trisomy 8 in patients with AML,[71] and, in the same year, Ruutu et al.[72] showed that neutrophils lacking a number 7 are defective in several granulocyte functions.[59] A year later, Borgström and associates[73] reported that patients whose leukemia cells are missing a number 7 have more infections and more temperature elevations than patients with a normal number of chromosomes.[59]

Rowley et al. (1977)[74] and Rowley (1978)[75] reported chromosomal abnormalities in patients with ANLL who had previously been treated for a different malignancy. Of 21 persons, 19 had lost all or part of chromosome 5 or 7 or both.[59] Keating and associates (1987), with a similar group of 32 patients who had a history of a prior malignancy or exposure to radiation or cytotoxic agents, found that 72 percent had an additional number 8 chromosome and/or loss or deletion of number 5 or 7. Only 8 percent of 351 patients without such a history had changes in chromosomes 5 or 7, or both.[76]

ALL

Acute lymphocytic leukemia occurs mainly in children, about 50 percent of whom attain long-term remissions and many of whom are now considered cured. The rest of the children and almost all adults survive briefly.[77] Progress in finding specific karyotypic alterations in this type of leukemia has been slower than in ANLL, and fewer large studies have been performed. Oshimura et al. (1977)[78] and Cimino et al. (1979)[79] found that about 50 percent of their patients who were investigated by banding had abnormal karyotypes.[59] Information from the Third International Workshop on Chromosomes in Leukemia (1981)[53] and a review article by Secker-Walker[77] show the following: (1) children whose malignant cells have more than 50 chromosomes have the best prognosis;[70] (2) patients with translocations have a poor prognosis, regardless of the chromosomes involved;[70] and (3) adults with 47 to 50 chromosomes have the worst prognosis of all.[77]

Three translocations, t(8;14)(q24;q32), t(2;8)(p12;q24), and t(8;22)(q24;q11), are associated with B cell neoplasia. They occur in leukemias and lymphomas (especially Burkitt's), and by far the most common is the t(8;14).[80] Chromosome 8q24 contains the c-*myc* protooncogene, whereas 14q32 is the site of an immunoglobulin heavy chain gene.[80,81] C-*myc* is translocated to the immunoglobulin locale in t(8;14); in the other two translocations, t(2;8) and t(8;22), c-*myc* remains on the derivative chromosome 8 but has parts of the immunoglobulin light-chain loci translocated into its immediate vicinity.[80] (Immunoglobulins act as specific antibodies and are found in numerous body fluids and tissues. At the molecular level, each immunoglobulin is composed of two light chains and two heavy chains, and this primary four-chain unit is repeated in immunoglobulins of high molecular weight.)

Thus, the adjacency of a known transforming gene (c-*myc*) and an immunoglobulin gene is implicated in some manner with a changed oncogene protein that is associated with malignant transformation.[65] The specific role that the c-*myc* protein plays in normal cells is still obscure.[82]

Williams et al. (1984) described a nonrandom translocation seen in pre-B-cell ALL in which most of the long arm of chromosome 1 is translocated to the short arm of number 19, t(1;19)(q23;p13.3).[83] A cellular oncogene, c-*ski*, is located at 1q23, and the insulin receptor gene is found at 19p13. It is not known whether rearrangement of these loci occurs in this translocation.[80]

The first description of a patient with ALL and a Ph[1] chromosome, t(9;22)(q34;q11), was that of Propp and Lizzi in 1970,[84] and other reports followed within a few years.[85–87]

Rowley delineated two types of Ph[1]-positive ALL, and, to differentiate, chromosome studies should be done while the patient is in remission: (1) Ph[1] ALL in which the karyotype becomes normal and (2) CML presenting in lymphoid blast crisis in which the karyotype remains essentially 100 percent Ph[1] positive.[59]

The Ph[1] chromosome may be the single most frequent cytogenetic rearrangement in ALL and is more often seen in adult patients than in children.[80] It has been detected in approximately 17 to 25 percent of adult patients who have ALL.[53,88,89] For patients with a specific rearrangement, such as t(9;22) or t(8;14), the survival curves in children and adults are virtually identical.[65] Is the Ph[1] chromosome in ALL identical at the molecular level with that seen in patients with CML? During January and February 1987, three relevant publications appeared.[88,90,91] Some patients who have ALL and the Ph chromosome translocation have the *bcr* rearrangement, and some do not. The cells of patients having the *bcr* rearrangement contain a phosphoprotein of relative molecular mass 210,000 (210K) called p210, which is the appropriate size for the *bcr-abl* fusion protein. In contrast, a phosphoprotein of 190K (p190) was seen in patients having the Ph chromosome but not the *bcr* rearrangement.[90] The authors suggested that the acute lymphoblastic leukemias having the *bcr-abl* chimeric gene coding p210 are probably lymphoid blast crises following a clinically silent CML; p190 cases are de novo acute lymphoblastic leukemias.[88,90,91]

Pinkel wrote that "cytogenetic features appear to influence remission duration and cure rate in many types of acute leukemia. While early pre-B ALL with hyperdiploidy has a high cure rate,[92] children who have a Ph chromosome in association with this same morphology and immunophenotype usually die of their disease."[93-95]

Several translocations, all involving chromosome 14q11, have been associated with T cell neoplasms, frequently T cell ALL. The 14q11 band contains the T cell receptor alpha-chain locus, and the translocations bring together protooncogenes and T cell receptor loci. This step may play a part in initiating these neoplasms.[80]

CLL, CML

In CLL, a low mitotic index has hindered cytogenetic analysis but, when cultures have been stimulated with B cell mitogens, chromosomal aberrations have been detected in more than 50 percent of patients with B cell CLL.[65,80] Trisomy 12 is seen in about one third of all patients who have CLL, and it has been suggested that this abnormality connotes a poor prognosis.[65] About 25 percent of patients show a 14q+ chromosome in which ma terial has been translocated to 14q32 from any one of a number of different chromosomes. According to Heim and Mitelman, "In some of these rearrangements, the immunoglobulin heavy chain locus in 14q32 has been shown to be split by the rearrangement, underscoring the principal similarity between these B cell abnormalities and the Burkitt-associated translocations."[80]

Rearrangements involving 14q11 are a feature of the more unusual T cell CLL, with inv(14)(q11q32) being found in one third of all cytogenetically abnormal T cell CLLs.[80]

The role of the Ph[1] chromosome in CML was reviewed in chapter 2.

EVALUATION

Dewald and associates (1985) commented that,

although the field of cytogenetics is rapidly evolving, it is clearly too early to depend completely on chromosome analysis for the diagnosis and classification of lymphomas and leukemias. Primarily because of technical problems and also biologic factors, identification of a chromosomally abnormal clone in all patients with malignant hematologic disorders is not always possible even though one may actually be present. In our experience, at the time of initial diagnosis the following proportions of patients with various hematologic disorders have a chromosomally abnormal clone on routine cytogenetic analysis: ANLL 54%, ALL 41%, CGL 94%, myelodysplastic syndrome 39%, and lymphoma 39%.[96]

In 1980, Sandberg stated that, "at present, there is no absolute evidence that a visibly recognizable karyotypic abnormality, with the possible exception of the Ph[1] in CML, plays a direct role in the causation of human cancer or leukemia."[3] He cited one case of the appearance of a Ph[1] in a patient with CML who had previously been Ph[1] negative, indicating that the induction of the Ph[1] was secondary to the CML,[3] and continued:

In addition, at least 50% of subjects with acute leukemia do not
have cytogenetic changes in their
leukemic cells, indicating that the
development of the leukemic state
does not necessarily have to be associated with an abnormal karyotypic picture. . . .

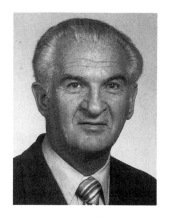

When one considers that the
average chromosome band con-
tains 5×10^6 base pairs and that a
deletion or duplication of 1/3 of a
band would be difficult if not impossible to detect with current

Avery A. Sandberg

methods [1980], it is premature, in my opinion, to correlate
such gross chromosomal changes, observed with the best of
banding techniques, with causation of neoplasia in human
subjects.[3]

When contacted in 1989, Sandberg updated his comments:

What has happened since 1980 has been the demonstration
that a significant number of leukemias, lymphomas and solid
tumors are associated with a microscopically visible and recurrent chromosomal change. This change, for example the
t(9;22)(q34;q11) leading to the Ph chromosome, may in a few
cases be directly responsible for the development of the leukemia, though this has not been proven. More and more tumors are being shown to be characterized by loss of genetic
material which cannot be ascertained cytogenetically and can
only be shown by molecular techniques. This tends to support
my statement of 1980 that in many cancers and leukemias the
chromosome changes, though they may be complex and/or
numerous, are epiphenomena secondary to the primary event
which is submicroscopic in nature. This is particularly true
of epithelial adenocarcinomas such as the most common cancers (e.g., tumors of the breast, lung, colon, bladder, prostate,
ovary and others).

Incidentally, the secondary (additional) chromosome changes,
though they are probably not related causally to the neoplasia,

must play a crucial role in its biology (metastatic spread, response to therapy, invasion). (A. A. Sandberg, personal communication, October 1989)

ONCOGENES

In addition to the chromosomal divergences just described in which whole chromosomes or sections of chromosomes are altered, other chromosome-related events have been identified in persons with cancer. It has been determined, for example, that certain genes with a potential for cancer may be positioned at breakpoints of some of the abnormal chromosomes. Also, some genes in normal cells seem to be analogous to viral oncogenes, the transforming genes of cancer-causing RNA tumor viruses called retroviruses. The cellular forms of the genes are called protooncogenes. By 1983, about two dozen protooncogenes had been discovered.[97] Because they seem to be universal, existing in all mammalian species thus far examined, in fruit flies, and even in yeast cells, scientists believe their function is so crucial that it has been perpetuated throughout evolution. They are believed to be involved in normal growth and differentiation.[98] It seems that the oncogenes of retroviruses "are miscreant copies of 'protooncogenes' or 'cellular oncogenes.' "[99]

J. Michael Bishop and Harold E. Varmus shared a Nobel Prize in medicine (1989) for their discovery of the cellular origin of retroviral oncogenes.[100] One of the first oncogenes isolated was the *src* (sarcoma) gene from the Rous sarcoma virus. This gene is responsible for cellular transformation but not virus replication.[101] Historically, this sarcoma virus is important because it was the first tumor virus to be studied seriously and it eventually became the most useful of the retroviruses.[102] It was found in 1911 by Francis Peyton Rous, working at the Rockefeller Institute.[103] He was awarded a Nobel Prize 55 years later (1966) at the age of 87; he was still working at that time.

Often, the oncogene is named after the virus from which it was first isolated. The *abl* oncogene (Abelson murine leukemia virus), located on chromosome 9, was discussed in chapter 2 in relation to CML. The *myc* oncogene (avian myelocytomatosis virus or acute leukemia virus MC 29) is located at the chromosomal breaks seen in leukemias and lymphomas, in particular in Burkitt's lymphoma. In humans, it is on chromosome 8. The *sis* oncogene (simian sarcoma virus), located on human chromosome 22, is also involved in the translocation seen in CML. The *ras*[H] oncogene (Harvey rat sarcoma virus), associated with Wilms' tumor, is on chromosome 11.[98]

In general, cellular oncogenes encode for proteins, and it would be a major advance if these proteins could be characterized. This has been difficult because they make up only a minute fraction of all proteins in the cell.[99] The available information shows "striking similarities (but never complete identity) between viral and cellular forms of the proteins."[99]

Also, it seems that the same oncogene may be active in different tumor types, e.g., "the cancer gene present within the DNA of lung cancer cells cannot be distinguished from that found within the DNA of colon cancer cells."[104]

As Bishop (1983) explained:

> The genes responsible for transformation of rodent cells by tumor DNA are being identified at a steady pace, and virtually all have come from within the *ras* family of cellular oncogenes. The identifications represent a considerable variety of tumors, including carcinomas of the colon, lung, pancreas, urinary bladder and gallbladder; neuroblastoma; and rhabdomyosarcoma. The reiterative appearance of cellular *ras* on this proscenium is provocative (some would say troubling) but presently inexplicable.[99]

Weinberg suggested that "maybe the oncogenes of the animal genome will be boiled down to a very small number of distinct types. Maybe the present oncogene jungle is not so impenetrable after all."[105]

Although experts warn that it is unlikely that the action of cellular oncogenes alone will prove to be the cause of neoplasia,[99] a less complicated overview of cancer may be on the horizon. As Bishop suggested, "a common set of cellular genes may help to mediate the genesis of all tumors, whatever their cause."[99]

NINE

Recombinant DNA and Human Molecular Analysis

It wasn't until the Nobel Prize
that they really thawed out.
They couldn't understand my work,
but they could understand $30,000.

WILLIAM FAULKNER (1897–1962), Quoted in *The National Observer*

In discussing human cytogenetics, we have been concerned with those components of the cell that relate to heredity, namely, the 46 chromosomes. However, scientists can now search deeper than the chromosome level: molecular geneticists examine molecules of DNA containing genes that, in humans, may number approximately 100,000. Although our primary interests are the medical applications of recombinant DNA technology and the potential for gene manipulation in leukemic disorders, a brief background describing the steps in the discovery of DNA and defining the techniques for genetic alterations should help us understand the remarkable achievements of our time.

EARLY GENETIC RESEARCH

Miescher

According to Chargaff,[1] Friedrich Miescher, living somewhere between Tübingen and Basel, discovered the nucleic acids in 1869.

His research was with nuclei of lymphocytes and, later, with spermatozoa from Rhine salmon. He succeeded in isolating deoxyribonucleic acid, which we now know as DNA.[2] Chargaff believes that Miescher was well aware of the importance of his work, as evidenced by his correspondence and his papers. Soon after Miescher's discovery of DNA, a description of ribonucleic acid (RNA) came from the laboratory of Hoppe-Seyler in Tübingen.[1]

Escherich

In 1885, when a German pediatrician, Theodor Escherich, isolated a species of bacteria from human feces,[3] he could never have foreseen the extent and detail of research to which it would be subjected nor the magnitude of the service it would render. The bacterium was named *Escherichia coli*, and it has been especially important in genetics research. In the 1940s, a small group of scientists agreed to use *E. coli*, whenever possible, to standardize their genetic experimentation, and that plan has been very successful and has contributed significantly to the rapid progress in molecular genetics.[4] Fortunately, some strains of *E. coli* are nonpathogenic and therefore very safe for laboratory use; also, because bacteria (and viruses) reproduce in 20 to 40 minutes, many offspring can be obtained in a day.

Griffith

Fred Griffith (1928) inadvertently made the next contribution to genetic research. While he was studying the bacteria (pneumococci) that cause various types of pneumonia, he found that some with rough coats (R variety) caused no disease when they were injected into mice, whereas others with smooth coats (S group) killed the mice. Griffith described in detail numerous lengthy experiments from which he learned that mice receiving simultaneous injections of nonpathogenic R cells from *Pneumococcus* type II and heat-killed type III (S) cells sometimes died of infection; when that happened, the virulent type III was recovered in blood culture.[5] Avery et al. later wrote:

> The fact that the R strain was avirulent and incapable by itself of causing fatal bacteremia and the additional fact that the heated suspension of Type III cells contained no viable organ-

isms brought convincing evidence that the R forms growing under these conditions had newly acquired the capsular structure and biological specificity of Type III pneumococci. . . .

. . . [Griffith had] succeeded in transforming an attenuated and non-encapsulated (R) variant derived from one specific type into fully encapsulated and virulent (S) cells of a heterologous specific type.[6]

Griffith had observed, without realizing it, a change in the DNA of some of the R cells that could then be bequeathed to all succeeding generations. The factor implementing this change was not destroyed by heat and, when it was assimilated into the R cells, could command them to make the capsule that was associated with virulence.[4]

According to Pollock, Griffith was a very modest and retiring person who preferred working quietly in his laboratory, rarely attending scientific meetings. A colleague reported that Griffith had to be practically forced into a taxi to go to the London International Microbiology Congress in 1936. He reluctantly read his paper in such a soft, unenthusiastic manner that those not closely concerned with the detailed streptococcal typing techniques must have been bored. It was the only paper he ever delivered at an open meeting, and it had nothing to do with transformation.[7]

1940 TO 1950

Avery

Oswald Avery was a contemporary of Griffith, although, as far as their associates knew, they never met. Avery and co-workers continued studying the pneumococcus, working to separate and identify the active component that took part in its transformation. Scientists had long supposed that genetic characteristics were related to the protein of the chromosomes, but the report of Avery et al. helped to center attention on nucleic acids.[8] They wrote:

The data obtained by chemical, enzymatic, and serological analyses together with the results of preliminary studies by electrophoresis, ultracentrifugation, and ultraviolet spectroscopy indicate that, within the limits of the methods, the active fraction contains no demonstrable protein, unbound lipid, or serologically reactive polysaccharide and consists principally, if not solely, of a highly polymerized, viscous form of desoxyribonucleic acid. . . .

. . . a nucleic acid of the desoxyribose type is the fundamental unit of the transforming principle of *Pneumococcus* Type III.[6]

Oswald Avery was not a big man physically—he weighed less than 100 pounds[9]—but he led his associates in a major discovery, and many believe he should have won a Nobel prize. At the time of his discovery, Avery, in a letter to his brother, wrote that the transforming agent "is in all probability DNA: who could have guessed it?"[7]

Pauling

In 1949, Linus Pauling and colleagues reported some of their genetic research on sickle cell anemia. They showed that a change occurring in a single gene led to the generation of an altered protein in hemoglobin molecules. As they explained:

In the chromosomes of a single nucleus of a normal adult somatic cell there is a complete absence of the sickle cell gene, while two doses of its allele are present; in the sicklemia somatic cell there exists one dose of each allele; and in the sickle cell anemia somatic cell there are two doses of the sickle cell gene, and a complete absence of its normal allele. Correspondingly, the erythrocytes of these individuals contain 100 percent normal hemoglobin, 40 percent sickle cell anemia hemoglobin and 60 percent normal hemoglobin, and 100 percent sickle cell anemia hemoglobin, respectively. This investigation reveals, therefore, a clear case of a change produced in a protein molecule by an allelic change in a single gene involved in synthesis.[10]

Pauling received the Nobel Prize for chemistry in 1954 for work on chemical bonds and molecular structure. When he was awarded the Peace Prize in 1962, he became the first person to receive two unshared Nobel Prizes in two different fields.

As a general rule, amino acids occur only in living tissue. Although, presumably, undetermined numbers of amino acids are possible, most proteins in living organisms are formed from various combinations and ratios of only 20 amino acids. Furthermore, whether amino acids are identified in a virus, an oak tree, a starfish, or a human, the same 20 (with rare exceptions) are present.[11] Amino acids are linked together into chains, generally one chain for each protein. Some proteins, however, consist of combinations of chains with different sequences of amino acids.[4]

Sanger

Sanger (1949) reported that the insulin molecule is composed of two amino acid chains: *A* is found in the more acidic fraction of oxidized insulin, contains glycine terminal residues, but has no arginine, histidine, lysine, phenylalanine, or threonine; *B* is the more basic fraction, contains phenylalanine terminal residues, and includes all of the amino acids present in insulin.[12]

Using methods for fractionating peptides on paper chromatograms, Sanger and Tuppy described the complete amino acid sequence in the phenylalanyl chain in 1951,[13,14] and 2 years later Sanger and Thompson determined the amino acid sequence in the glycyl chain. They subjected the more acidic fraction of oxidized insulin to partial hydrolysis and fractionated the resulting peptides by charcoal adsorption, iontophoresis, and paper chromatography.[15] Frederick Sanger was awarded the Nobel Prize in chemistry (1958) in recognition of these accomplishments.

1950 TO 1960

Chargaff

In 1950, Chargaff's landmark paper, "Chemical Specificity of Nucleic Acids and Mechanism of their Enzymatic Degradation," appeared in *Experientia*. In it he stated that

the desoxypentose nucleic acids from animal and microbial cells contain varying proportions of the same four nitrogenous constituents, namely adenine [A], guanine [G], cytosine [C], thymine [T]. Their composition appears to be characteristic of the species, but not of the tissue, from which they are derived.

The presumption, therefore, is that there exists an enormous number of structurally different nucleic acids. . . .

If [the nucleic acid] consists of 2,500 nucleotides, . . . then the number of possible "isomers" is not far from 10^{1500}. . . .

. . . as far as chemical possibilities go, [nucleic acids] could very well serve as one of the agents, or possibly as the agent, concerned with the transmission of inherited properties.[16]

In 1951, Chargaff explained further that two principal categories of DNA are apparent, the *AT type* in which adenine and thymine dominate, and the *GC type* in which guanine and cytosine are the major components. Also, "in almost all DNA preparations studied, the ratio of total purines to total pyrimidines never was far from 1. Similarly, the ratios of adenine to thymine and of guanine to cytosine were near 1."[17]

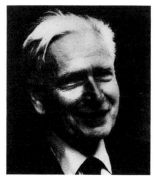

Erwin Chargaff

Brown and Todd

At about the same time, Brown and Todd were studying the chemistry of nucleic acids and of nucleotides. The latter are compounds composed of a base (purine or pyrimidine), a sugar (ribose or deoxyribose), and a phosphate group. In a 1952 publication, they stated that "there can be no doubt that $C_{(5')}$ is involved in the main internucleotide linkage both of ribonucleic and of deoxyribonucleic acids. In the case of the latter, the main linkage must be the $C_{(3')} - C_{(5')}$, but a decision between $C_{(2')}$ and $C_{(3')}$ as the second point of attachment in ribonucleic acids cannot yet be made with certainty."[18] Their article included a diagram of their conception of the backbone structure of nucleic acids.

Both DNA and RNA are polydiesters of phosphoric acid in which the individual nucleotides are linked in a uniform, linear manner.[8] The DNA nucleotide is the phosphate ester of the sugar 2-deoxy-D-ribofuranose linked to one of four bases: adenine, guanine, cytosine, or thymine.[8,19] The first three bases are also used in RNA, but thymine appears only in DNA; it is replaced by a similar pyrimidine, uracil, in RNA.

D'Herelle

In 1948, Delbrück and Delbrück stated that bacterial viruses were first discovered about 30 years previously by the French bacteriologist F. D'Herelle,[20,21] who noticed that bacteria growing in some of his test tubes mysteriously dissolved. "After experimentation D'Herelle concluded that their dissolution was due to some agent much smaller than a bacterium, and that this agent grew at the expense of bacteria. He called the agents that had destroyed the bacteria 'bacteriophage' (bacteria-eaters): the same organisms are now often called bacterial viruses."[22]

Hershey and Chase

By the late 1930s, scientists working with bacterial viruses had learned how to infect bacteria with virus particles. When a virus particle attaches to a bacterial cell wall, the viral DNA enters the cell and the virus multiplies very rapidly. Hershey and Chase reported what they had learned from studying T2 (a bacteriophage that infects *E. coli*), in 1953: "One of the first steps in the growth of T2 is the release from its protein coat of the nucleic acid of the virus particle. . . . when a particle of bacteriophage T2 attaches to a bacterial cell, most of the phage DNA enters the cell, and a residue containing at least 80 per cent of the sulfur-containing protein of the phage remains at the cell surface."[23] Their work really settled the question of whether genetic characteristics were carried in a protein or solely in DNA.

Alfred Hershey, Max Delbrück, and Salvador Luria were Nobel laureates in 1969 in recognition of their pioneer studies with the phages of *E. coli*. Delbrück and his associates chose to work on T-even phages, whose best host is *E. coli*; their research contributed further to the extensive use of that bacterium in research.

Pauling and Corey

In 1953, the truly milestone articles on the structure of DNA appeared in the British journal *Nature*. In the issue of February 21st, Pauling and Corey wrote on nucleic acids:

The structure involves three intertwined helical polynucleotide chains. Each chain which is formed by phosphate di-ester
groups and linking β-D-ribofuranose or β-D-deoxyribofuranose
residues with 3′, 5′ linkages, has approximately twenty-four
nucleotide residues in seven turns of the helix. The helixes
have the sense of a right-handed screw. The phosphate groups
are closely packed about the axis of the molecule, with the
pentose residues surrounding them, and the purine and pyrimidine groups projecting radially, their planes being approximately perpendicular to the molecular axis.[24]

Watson and Crick

On April 25, 1953, Watson and Crick, stating that the Pauling
and Corey manuscript had been made available to them before it
appeared in print, presented their theory.

We wish to put forward a radically different structure for the
salt of deoxyribose nucleic acid. This structure has two helical
chains each coiled around the same axis. We have made the
usual chemical assumptions, namely that each chain consists
of phosphate diester groups joining β-D-deoxyribofuranose residues with 3′,5′ linkages. . . .
  The novel feature of the structure is the manner in which
the two chains are held together by the purine and pyrimidine
bases. The planes of the bases are perpendicular to the fibre
axis. They are joined together in pairs, a single base from one
chain being hydrogen-bonded to a single base from the other
chain. . . . if an adenine forms one member of a pair, on either
chain, then on these assumptions the other member must be
thymine; similarly for guanine and cytosine.[25]

In the same issue of *Nature* an account by Wilkins et al. described their x-ray diffraction studies of deoxypentose nucleic
acids.[26] Their diffraction photographs had been available to Watson and Crick.

Kornberg

The next major contribution to DNA research came from
Kornberg and colleagues (1956). They discovered DNA polymer-

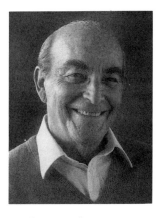

Arthur Kornberg

ase, an enzyme that activates the union of nucleotides into DNA chains.[27,28] Polymerase enzymes catalyze polymerization, the process of forming a high-molecular-weight compound by combining simpler molecules. As Kornberg remembered:

> My colleagues and I first undertook to synthesize nucleic acids outside the living cell, with the help of cellular enzymes, in 1954. . . . We attained our goal within a year, but not until . . . 14 years later were we able to report a completely synthetic DNA, made with natural DNA as a template, that has the full biological activity of the native material. . . .

In our first attempts to achieve DNA synthesis in a cell-free system we used the deoxyribonucleoside called deoxythymidine. . . . We were hopeful that extracts of *E. coli* would be able to incorporate deoxythymidine into nucleic acid by converting it first into the 5′ deoxynucleotide and then activating the deoxynucleotide to the triphosphate form. I found this to be the case. . . .

In November 1955, I. Robert Lehman . . . started on the purification of the enzyme system in *E. coli* extracts that is responsible for converting deoxythymidine 5′-triphosphate into DNA. We were joined by Maurice J. Bessman some weeks later. Those were eventful days in which the enzyme, now given the name DNA polymerase, was progressively separated from other large molecules. With each step in purification the character of this DNA synthetic reaction became clearer.[29]

Lwoff

About the same time (1953) André Lwoff showed that phage DNA could multiply in the cytoplasm of a bacterium or could implant itself in the chromosome of the bacterium and perform in a manner similar to that of the authentic bacterial genes. The latter was termed a *prophage* form, a word originated by Lwoff and a co-worker, Antoinette Gutmann.[30] During the prophage interval, the bacterium is "lysogenic," "possessing and transmitting the power to produce bacteriophage."[30] Lwoff explained:

> In order that a bacterium may become lysogenic, the genetic material of the infecting phage has to be attracted and bound to a specific chromosomal receptor. Prophage thus appears not only as a specific structure but a specific structure localized at a specific site. . . .
> Lysogenic bacteria survive only if prophage does not develop into phage. In lysogenic bacteria, a reaction must be blocked which is necessary for the development of prophage. As a matter of fact, in lysogenic bacteria the infecting homologous and related phages are also unable to develop. This is immunity.[30]

In a subsequent lecture, Lwoff noted that, "when a phage infects a bacterium, two possibilities are open. Either the genetic material of the phage enters the vegetative phase of the cycle and phage is produced, or it becomes attached to the bacterial chromosome and is transformed into a prophage. . . . Prophage is the genetic material of the phage as modified by its binding to the bacterial chromosome."[31]

Meselson and Stahl

Meselson and Stahl (1958) reported that "studies of bacterial transformation and bacteriophage infection strongly indicate that DNA can carry and transmit hereditary information and can direct its own replication."[32] Their brilliant experiments showed that, in replication, the two strands of the double helix unwind, and each single strand acts as a template for a new daughter double helix.[4,32]

Todd

Lord Alexander Todd gave a lecture at the Royal Society of Medicine in 1959 and pointed out that research with bacterial viruses documented very strongly that genetic continuity resides in the DNA.

Infection of the host cells is accomplished through injection of phage DNA; the protein coat remains outside and at most only very small amounts of protein enter the host. . . .

The evidence available . . . shows clearly that nucleic acids can and do act as genes or carriers of genetic information, and it is at least highly probable that they do so in all forms of living matter and in the viruses.[19]

Todd expressed hope that research with bacterial viruses could lead to effective cancer therapy. The *British Medical Journal* (1959) quoted him as saying: "Agents which interfered with base-pairing might well destroy a virus or render it harmless; they might equally lead to the destruction of the cancer cell . . . a rational approach to the chemotherapy of virus diseases and of cancer could be made. A long series of purine and pyrimidine antagonists have been made—substances like 6-MP and 5-FU have shown promise."[33] If chemotherapy were going to be more than a hit-or-miss affair, however, Todd believed that success must be achieved in two areas: (1) pure individual nucleic acids must be prepared and (2) ways must be found to study their structure and clarify their relationships to one another.[19]

1960 TO 1970

Monod and Jacob

Jacques Monod and François Jacob studied techniques regulating the construction and the quantity of proteins within the cell. Their extensive research characterized the beta-galactosidase enzyme and its role as a catalyst and revealed that inducers and repressors control the synthesis of messenger RNA. In a subsequent review article they stated that

the synthesis of enzymes in bacteria follows a double genetic control. The so-called structural genes determine the molecular organization of the proteins. Other, functionally specialized, genetic determinants, called regulator and operator genes, control the rate of protein synthesis through the intermediacy of cytoplasmic components or repressors. The repressors can be either inactivated (induction) or activated (repression) by certain specific metabolites. This system of regulation appears to operate directly at the level of the synthesis by the gene of a short-lived intermediate, or messenger, which becomes associated with the ribosomes where protein synthesis takes place.[34]

Nobel Prizes

The decades of the 1950s and 1960s were very prolific periods for researchers in molecular biology and related fields, and, subsequently, their accomplishments were acknowledged with many Nobel Prizes. Lord Alexander Todd received the Nobel Prize in chemistry in 1957, and Joshua Lederberg and Edward Tatum were recipients in physiology or medicine in 1958. Lederberg was lauded "for his discoveries concerning genetic recombination and the organization of the genetic material of bacteria."[35] His studies with *E. coli* showed that, in some cases, bacteria were sexual. Tatum was rewarded for "discovering that genes act by regulating specific chemical processes."[35] He had worked with George Beadle, and, "even before the big discoveries of the 1950s, they had figured out from mold research that a single gene codes for a single enzyme."[9] Arthur Kornberg was a Nobel winner in 1959. His fundamental work on nucleotides "led to his landmark discovery that nucleotides line up on one strand of nucleic acid to form another strand with a complementary nucleotide sequence."[36]

In 1962, Watson, Crick, and Wilkins were named Nobel laureates in physiology or medicine; today, Watson is in charge of the genome project. The 1965 prize in physiology or medicine was bestowed on the three French biologists, Lwoff, Jacob, and Monod, for their contributions to the accumulated knowledge of gene functions.

The 1968 Nobel Prize for physiology or medicine was awarded to Marshall Nirenberg of the NIH, Har Gobind Khorana of the University of Wisconsin, and Robert Holley, previously at Cornell University, all prominent for work deciphering the genetic code.

Nirenberg and Matthaei

By 1953, it was known that DNA did not directly instruct amino acids to make protein. Such a concept seemed unreasonable because most DNA is found in the nucleus, and protein synthesis takes place in the cytoplasm.[4] An intermediary must exist to transfer information from the DNA to the cytoplasm, where it could direct the sequence of amino acids in synthesizing a protein. As soon as the double helix was discovered, RNA became the primary suspect. Watson et al. explained:

> For one thing, the cytoplasm of cells that made large numbers of proteins always contained large amounts of RNA. Even more importantly, the sugar-phosphate backbones of DNA and RNA were known to be quite similar, and it was easy to imagine the synthesis of single RNA chains upon single-stranded DNA templates to yield unstable hybrid molecules in which one strand was DNA and the other strand was RNA. Here it is important to note that the unique base of RNA, uracil, is chemically very similar to thymine in that it specifically base-pairs to adenine.[4]

Thus, a single DNA strand could be a template for complementary DNA (by replication) or for complementary RNA (by transcription). "In turn, the RNA molecules serve as the templates that order the amino acids within the polypeptide chains of proteins during the process of translation, so named because the nucleotide language of nucleic acids is translated into the amino acid language of proteins."[4] Although this pathway was established by 1961, there seemed no likelihood that the secrets of the genetic code would soon be solved.

In 1961, however, Nirenberg and Matthaei showed that protein synthesis occurs in cell-free extracts from bacterial cells.[37] In addition, "when synthetic RNAs of known composition are added to these cell free systems, they specify short proteins that can easily be analyzed. [Polyuridylic acid], an RNA containing only uracil, specified a protein containing only one amino acid, phenylalanine. The code word for phenylalanine must be a sequence of uracil residues."[38] In their original paper, Nirenberg and Matthaei reported that

> a stable, cell-free system [had] been obtained from *E. coli* in which the amount of incorporation of amino acids into protein was dependent upon the addition of heat-stable template RNA preparations. Soluble RNA could not replace template RNA fractions. . . .

> ... The function of ribosomal RNA remains an enigma, although at least part of the total RNA is thought to serve as templates for protein synthesis and has been termed "messenger" RNA.[37]

Within 5 years after that publication most of the code words had been assigned. These cited the amino acids involved but did not tell the sequence.

> For example, the code word for asparagine contains 2 As and 1 C, while that for histidine has 2 Cs and an A. But is the sequence of the histidine code word ... CCA, ACC, or CAC? Nirenberg found that by adding trinucleotides (single code words) to ribosomes, the amino acid specified by that code word was attached to the ribosome by its specific transfer RNA. Trinucleotides of known sequence are relatively simple to synthesize so that the order of code words was quickly determined.[38]

Khorana

Khorana (1960) attacked the problems of the chemical synthesis of polynucleotides.[39] He originated a way to make lengthy DNA or RNA molecules of ascertained sequence. He used DNA and RNA polymerase enzymes to make long molecules containing all 64 possible triplets (codons) of the four nucleic acid bases.[38] "He showed that triplets do not overlap and that in protein synthesis they are read in sequence without gaps between them."[36] By 1966, the genetic code was entirely solved: 61 of the 64 possible triplets coded for specific amino acids, and the other 3 coded for stop signals.[4]

Holley

Holley and colleagues were the first to report the exact nucleotide sequence of a nucleic acid. They chose the alanine transfer-RNA molecule of yeast because it is comparatively small, containing 77 nucleotides.[40,41] This transfer RNA "recognizes the amino acid alanine and transfers it to the site where it can be incorporated into a growing polypeptide chain. When such a chain assumes its final configuration, sometimes joining with other chains, it is called a protein."[42]

Holley later explained that the determination of the nucleotide sequence culminated 7 years of work by his group at Cornell University. They had broken the RNA chain by using two enzymes. The first severed the chain immediately to the right of pyrimidine nucleotides, producing a set of relatively long fragments. The second enzyme cut the chain specifically to the right of purine nucleotides, yielding somewhat shorter fragments. The fragments were sorted by passing them through a thin glass column packed with diethylaminoethyl cellulose; the short sections passed through the column more rapidly than did the long. The nucleotides in each fragment were released by hydrolyzing with an alkali. Then, the individual nucleotides were identified by paper chromatography, paper electrophoresis, and spectrographic analysis.[42] This is a very simplified version of their complex procedure.

As soon as Holley's sequence had been reported, Khorana started to synthesize the gene for yeast alanine transfer RNA. When he received the Nobel Prize, he described how half of the molecule had thus far been made.[38]

DNA Ligase

In 1967, another giant step was taken when five separate research groups described an enzyme that came to be known as DNA ligase.[43–47] This is a sealing enzyme that can repair nicks in DNA and can seal together fragments of DNA that have been cut from the strand.

In 1970, while Khorana's group was assembling the first synthetic gene, they found that the ligase from the T4 bacteriophage catalyzed the joining of DNA duplexes at their base-paired ends to yield products of higher molecular weight.[48] When DNA is cut, some enzymes produce segments that have blunt ends with no inclination to adhere to one another. Other enzymes yield segments with "tail" ends, and complementary single-stranded tails tend to come together by base pairing. The tails came to be called "sticky" ends. If two fragments of DNA could be stuck together, they could later be joined permanently by exposure to the DNA ligase enzyme.[4]

Smith and Wilcox

During the 1960, researchers realized that, to find the exact order of the bases (A, T, G, C) in a DNA molecule (in other words, to "sequence" the molecule), they would have to find a way to cut the long DNA filament into selected segments. Most enzymes that did break the bonds splintered the DNA into such small portions that their possible arrangement in the original strand could not be ascertained.[4] However, in 1970, Smith and Wilcox reported discovering the first restriction enzyme, an enzyme that split DNA at particular locations. They had incubated *Haemophilus influenzae* cells with radioactively labeled DNA from the *Salmonella* phage P22 and found that the

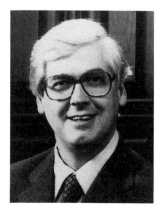

Hamilton O. Smith

DNA was apparently broken down (degraded). "We have been particularly interested in the ability of [the enzyme] endonuclease R to 'recognize' only a few specific sites on rather large foreign DNA molecules."[49]

Yoshimori

About the same time, another restriction enzyme, *Eco*RI, was identified by Yoshimori,[50] a graduate student at the University of California Medical School at San Francisco.[3] It was named *Eco* because it came from a strain of *E. coli*; R indicated that it resisted antibiotics. The *Eco*RI enzyme made zigzag cuts in the two DNA strands so that each resulting segment had a tail or sticky end.

Boyer

In the late 1960s, Boyer and Roulland-Dussoix were working on bacterial mechanisms for DNA restriction and modification. It was known that strains of *E. coli* have a means of rejecting nonhomologous DNA (e.g., DNA originating in a cell from a different strain).[51] As they explained:

> Bacteriophage, bacterial and episomal DNA, when transferred from *E. coli* K12 to *E. coli* B, or vice versa, are subject to host-

controlled restriction, or specific degradation by the recipient cell. This destruction is brought about by an endonuclease which introduces a limited number of double-strand scissions at defined sites along the DNA molecule. Intrastrain transfer of DNA is not subject to restriction because these sites are modified. This latter process is known as host-controlled modification of DNA.[51]

In 1971 Boyer reported that restriction and modification of bacterial DNA are not limited to certain strains of *E. coli* but are common in microorganisms. He identified at least two types of restriction and modification mechanisms and recognized that endonucleases and methylases are the enzymologic bases of both mechanisms. He concluded that "the various restriction endonucleases with exclusive recognition capacities offer a unique probe for dissecting small genomes."[52]

Further experiments (Boyer et al., 1973) with Eco_{RII} tended to show that both enzymes (restriction endonuclease and modification methylase) interacted with the same substrate, a specific sequence of nucleotide base pairs in double-stranded DNA.[53]

1970 TO 1980

Mertz and Davis

By the early 1970s, then, the stage was set, and the next decade became known for the remarkable achievements in developing techniques for genetic alteration. The first recombinant DNA molecules were synthesized at Stanford University (1972). Mertz used *Eco*RI to cut the circular DNA of the monkey virus SV40. She noted that the severed ends seemed to be trying to connect themselves back together again. Lear explained that Davis, using the electron microscope, was able to see the staggered or zigzag breaks in the DNA and to observe the tails or sticky ends.[3] Mertz and Davis found, in addition, that all DNA cleaved by *Eco*RI, regardless of origin, acquired sticky ends. They came to realize that any two DNA molecules cut by this method could be recombined by using DNA ligase. Thus, hybrid DNA molecules would be formed.[3] Mertz and Davis found that "R_I endonuclease, in conjunction with DNA ligase, provides a means for *in vitro*, site-specific recombination: Any two DNAs with R_I endonuclease cleavage sites can be 'recombined' at their restriction sites by the sequential action of R_I endonuclease and DNA ligase."[54] Other researchers at Stanford were working on the same problem of joining DNA molecules, and during 1971 and 1972 another method for recombining DNA molecules was devised by Lobban and Kaiser[55] and by Jackson, Symons, and Berg.[56] Both used an enzyme called terminal transferase (described in 1967 by Kato et al.[57]) along with ligase to combine molecules.

Cohen

Plasmid is a general term for many types of intracellular inclusions that have genetic functions. Plasmids are DNA molecules capable of replicating, but they are separate from the primary DNA genome. Bacteria have chromosomes containing several million base pairs and, also, may have tiny, spherical plasmids with only several thousand base pairs.[4] Some plasmids encode antibiotic resistance and are called R-factors.[58]

Plasmid DNA is relatively easy to separate and purify. Cohen (Stanford) had isolated a plasmid from *E. coli* that he named R (resistant to antibiotics) 6-5. Lear explained that Cohen then separated a small piece of the DNA that he labeled Tc6-5 to signify that it was resistant only to tetracycline. This segment formed a ring and, itself, became a plasmid. When Tc6-5 was mixed with *Eco*RI, the midget plasmid was cleaved only once. It retained the genes for tetracycline resistance and for replication. It was named pSC (for Stanley Cohen) 101. Cohen and co-workers subsequently joined the DNA of pSC101 to the DNA of other plasmids derived from R6-5 and also to the DNA of other plasmids from organisms different from *E. coli.*[3]

Their work was significant for several reasons: (1) it introduced plasmids as vectors; (2) it used a strong marker (tetracycline resistance) so that the recombinant DNA could be easily detected after it had entered host plasmid-free bacterial cells, which are antibiotic-sensitive; (3) it was a simpler method than the virus hybridizing described by Jackson, Symons, and Berg; and (4) it provided the background for "the first complete recombinant DNA experiments in which foreign DNA was joined to pSC101 DNA in the test tube, introduced into *E. coli,* replicated many times, the DNA reisolated and studied, and finally, even the expression of functions by the recombinant DNA was studied in *E. coli.*"[58] The publications by Cohen and colleagues are of landmark importance.[59,60]

Asilomar Conferences

By 1971, some members of the scientific community had learned of the studies being pursued at Stanford that would join the DNA from the eukaryotic simian tumor virus 40 (SV40) to DNA of the prokaryotic lambda bacteriophage, which would then become a vector to transport the SV40 hybrid into *E. coli.* Eukaryotes are organisms whose cells have nuclei, and this category includes all plants and animals. Prokaryotes are organisms without a true nucleus, and the bacterial viruses (bacteriophage) are in this grouping. As far as the scientists were aware, nature had never allowed any exchange of genes between prokaryotes and eukaryotes. Some experts were uneasy about such gene splicing. In a letter to *Science*, Chargaff wrote, "Are we wise in getting ready to mix up what nature has kept apart, namely the genomes of eukaryotic and prokaryotic cells?"[61]

Knowledgeable persons realized that as soon as the SV40 hybrid was inside *E. coli*, it would "multiply as *E. coli* multiplied, once every twenty minutes."[3] As SV40 caused tumors in small animals, they were concerned that SV40 DNA might evade its keepers and become very dangerous to humans: "you cannot recall a new form of life. . . . Once you have constructed a viable *E. coli* carrying a plasmid DNA into which a piece of eukaryotic DNA has been spliced, it will survive you and your children and your children's children."[61] Therefore, for the first time in history, scientists, voluntarily, called an interim halt to certain areas of recombinant DNA experimentation.

One hundred invited delegates from the United States and one from England attended the first Asilomar Conference in California (January 1973) to discuss these concerns; subsequently, an international forum was held at the same site in February 1975.[3] The NIH directives that followed (July 1976) classified and controlled laboratories according to risk potential and limited some experimentation, particularly that with oncogenic viruses. These discussions and actions plus the misgivings of some scientists were reported by the media and led to public anxiety regarding the enforceability and adequacy of the NIH guidelines. A writer for the *New York Times Magazine* advocated forbidding the awarding of the Nobel Prize for recombinant DNA research. In 1979, however, the NIH decided that the fears had been exaggerated, and officials loosened the restrictions, allowing the study of cancer viruses to proceed.[3,4]

Fiers et al.

These researchers from the University of Ghent, Belgium, reported the entire nucleotide sequence of the bacteriophage MS2 RNA (1976). MS2 is, therefore, the first living organism for which the complete chemical constitution was described. The RNA is 3569 nucleotides long.[62] The same group, in a repeat performance (1978), unraveled the total 5224 base-pair DNA sequence of the virus SV40.[63]

Reverse Transcriptase

Howard Temin, Renato Dulbecco, and David Baltimore shared a Nobel Prize in 1975. Baltimore and Temin (with co-author Mizutani) had independently discovered an enzyme in virions of RNA tumor viruses that synthesized DNA from an RNA template. Apparently the transfer of information, which is usually from DNA to RNA, could occur also in reverse.[64] Their original articles appeared in the same issue of *Nature*,[65,66] and Baltimore's was the most-cited paper during the 10-year period after its publication. As the editor of *Nature* commented, their findings had "important implications not only for carcinogenesis by RNA viruses but also for the general understanding of genetic transcription."[64] Later studies verified the existence of the enzyme (reverse transcriptase).

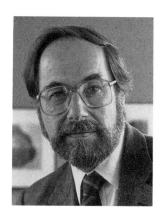

David Baltimore

Dulbecco contributed research on the role of viruses in cancer. He developed the first quantitative assay for infectious virus particles in animals.[67]

More Nobel Awards

Daniel Nathans, Hamilton Smith, and Werner Arber were Nobel recipients in 1978 for their contributions to the knowledge of
restriction enzymes. The prize in chemistry in 1980 went to Paul
Berg, Walter Gilbert, and Frederick Sanger. Gilbert and Sanger
were recognized for developing techniques for sequencing base-
pair fragments of DNA, Sanger using enzymes and Gilbert using
chemical degradation of DNA chains.[4] This was Sanger's second
Nobel award in chemistry. Among his many achievements, Sanger is noted also for finding two instances of genes located within
genes, previously thought to be impossible.[35] Berg, at Stanford,
was a pioneer in the development of recombinant DNA techniques for introducing new genetic information into mammalian
cells with virus DNA vectors. He described how DNA transfers
genetic information to RNA, which in turn creates new templates
for making new proteins.[36] He chaired both forums at the Asilomar Conference Center.

MEDICAL APPLICATIONS

Genetic engineering has created a new industrial complex called
biotech. Since around 1980, many of the advances in DNA research have emerged from the laboratories of these companies.
They can mass-produce many substances because they have learned
how to transform bacterial cells into small factories. When a
segment of foreign DNA is inserted into a plasmid (or other vector),
a hybrid plasmid containing recombinant DNA is created. When
these DNA molecules are introduced into host bacteria (or yeast),
they become part of the host DNA in some instances. Cells containing the recombinant DNA molecules can be identified and
separated if a marker (e.g., antibiotic resistance) exists. Because
the DNA strands separate and replicate every 20 to 40 minutes,
numerous exact copies, or clones, of that cell are produced. Each
of these clones has the capacity to formulate whatever the DNA
instructs it to prepare, and the selected substance can then be
segregated from the bacteria. This is a very simplified explanation
of the basic process, but each substance produced thus far by this
method represents a complex and remarkable genetic engineering

achievement. The expectation is that these end-products, usually proteins, can be volume-produced less expensively and in a more purified state by cloning.[4] In 1980, the Supreme Court justices ruled that the procedure for producing recombinant DNA could be patented.

Recombinant Somatostatin

Itakura and colleagues (1977) reported "the first success in achieving expression (that is, transcription into RNA and translation of that RNA into a protein of a designed amino acid sequence) of a gene of chemically synthesized origin."[68] They created somatostatin, the first human hormone produced by recombinant DNA technology. Somatostatin retards the secretion of several other hormones (growth hormone, insulin, glucagon) and may be of value in treating acromegaly, acute pancreatitis, and insulin-dependent diabetes.[68] Itakura et al. chose to work with somatostatin because of "its small size and known amino acid sequence."[68]

Recombinant Insulin

In 1979, Goeddel and coauthors described the "assembly and cloning of the genes for the A and B chains [of human insulin], their insertion into the . . . *E. coli* beta-galactosidase structural gene, the expression and purification of the separate A and B chains, and their joining to form native human insulin."[69] Recombinant insulin, marketed since 1982, is being used by diabetics, especially those who are allergic to or have unpleasant side effects from pig insulin.

Recombinant Human Growth Hormone

Also in 1979, Goeddel's group "designed and constructed a bacterial plasmid which instructs the synthesis of substantial quantities of mature human growth hormone in a microbial cell."[70] Human growth hormone consists of 191 amino acids and is made in the anterior lobe of the pituitary. Before the development of recombinant techniques, the only source was human cadavers. The limited supply was reserved for hypopituitary dwarfs whose growth can be stimulated if growth hormone is administered during childhood. A ready supply of recombinant hormone is now available for children of very short stature; it is administered also to children with cancer and "may prove effective in a variety of other ailments, including bone fractures, skin burns, and bleeding ulcers."[70] Goeddel et al. used a novel combination of chemically synthesized DNA and complementary DNA to construct a recombinant *E. coli* strain that produces human growth hormone in large amounts.[70] This was "the first time that a human polypeptide has been directly expressed in *E. coli* in a non-precursor form."[70]

Recombinant Interferon

The three types of human interferon (leukocyte, fibroblast, and immune) were discussed in chapter 7. During the 1970s, researchers working with the interferons had no knowledge of their amino acid sequences or the composition of their genes.[4] Therefore, cloning interferon genes did not seem imminent. There was special incentive to produce recombinant interferon, however, because the natural substance was in short supply and was very expensive and because leukocyte interferon isolated from human buffy-coat cells was only about 1 percent pure.[71] Progress in interferon research was delayed because of the limited quantity available.

Then, in 1979, Taniguchi and associates[72] described the construction and identification of a bacterial plasmid containing cloned sequences that hybridized specifically to human fibroblast interferon messenger RNA.[73] As Yelverton and Goeddel stated, "Subsequently, Taniguchi et al. (1980)[74] and workers in Belgium (1980)[75,76] and the United States (1980)[77] have identified and sequenced cloned complementary DNA copies of fibroblast interferon messenger RNA, and have achieved bacterial expression of the complementary DNA genes."[73]

In 1980, Nagata's group in Switzerland reported "the isolation of a hybrid plasmid containing an 872-base pair leukocyte-interferon complementary DNA, which elicits the information in *Escherichia coli*, of a polypeptide with the immunological and biological properties of human leukocyte-interferon."[78] That same year, Secher and Burke of the United Kingdom described the production of a monoclonal antibody to human leukocyte interferon. The antibody could be used for large-scale purification of interferon, allowing purification up to 5,000-fold in a single step.[79]

Molecular cloning of human immune interferon complementary DNA and its expression in eukaryotic cells was reported (1982) by a group at Genentech, Inc., in California[80] and also by researchers at the University of Ghent, Belgium.[81]

Since these successes in cloning the interferon genes, commercial production has supplied sufficient amounts of interferon for research and testing in a variety of diseases. Researchers at Hoffmann-LaRoche, Inc., used leukocytes from M. D. Anderson Cancer Center patients with CML for a supply of crude alpha-interferon to begin their task of purification in 1977. By January 1981, they had supplied recombinant interferon A (as they designated it) to Gutterman at M. D. Anderson Cancer Center for the first clinical trial in cancer patients.[82] The early studies in the leukemias have been outlined in chapter 7.

It now seems preferable to designate the classes of interferons as alpha, beta, and gamma rather than as leukocyte, fibroblast, and immune because a single cell type may make more than one class of interferon. For example, a plasmid whose messenger RNA had been synthesized in leukocytes was found to carry the DNA sequence coding for a human beta (fibroblast) interferon.[82]

In recent years, other biologic response modifiers (GM-CSF, interleukin 1, interleukin 2, human tumor necrosis factor) have been synthesized using recombinant DNA techniques.

Sickle-Cell Anemia

This was the first genetic disease to be diagnosed before birth by restriction enzyme analysis of DNA (1978).[83] Watson et al.[4] stated that by 1983 more than 40 disorders could be determined antenatally. When genetic disorders are identified, parents may select abortion for a fetus facing a hopeless future. It is anticipated that human gene manipulation (the insertion of normal genes to replace abnormal ones) may become possible in the not-too-distant future.

1980 TO 1990

Recently (January 1989), scientists at the Lawrence Livermore Laboratory in California using a scanning tunneling electron microscope saw, for the first time, a molecule of DNA.[84] When magnified up to 1,000,000 times, the double helix is visible to the eye. The molecule coils as Watson and Crick described, and it is possible to measure the distance between successive coils, about 1/5,500,000th of an inch.[85]

In the spring of 1989, researchers at the National Institutes of Health transplanted a foreign gene into a human for the first time. Tumor-infiltrating lymphocytes were removed from a patient with a very advanced melanoma, tagged with neomycin resistance by inserting an altered mouse virus gene so that the lymphocytes could be traced, cultured with IL-2, and allowed to multiply. The cells were then returned to the patient, and the researchers expect that the tagging will help them determine whether these special cancer-fighting cells arrive at the tumor location and have a positive effect.[86,87]

In September 1989, Francis Collins (University of Michigan Medical Center) and Lap-Chee Tsui (Hospital for Sick Children in Toronto), after studying material from 54 families that included members with cystic fibrosis, were able to place the cystic fibrosis gene on chromosome 7.[88]

CONCLUDING REMARKS

At present, most of the material in this chapter may seem irrelevant to leukemia, but we believe that molecular genetics has already assumed a major role in the study of this disorder.

We were unable to find any publication that reviewed in a step-by-step sequence the discoveries that culminated in recombinant DNA techniques. Therefore, in this chapter we have attempted a brief summary, endeavoring to simplify descriptions of complex experimental research that is often bewildering to readers outside the field.

Recombinant interferon is now used for patients who have hairy cell leukemia, CML in the chronic phase, and some myeloproliferative disorders; recombinant GM-CSF is used for the treatment of myelodysplasias and to treat the granulocytopenia accompanying chemotherapy or bone marrow transplantation. The use of recombinant products is expected to be widespread before long.

It is not unrealistic to foresee gene manipulation in families with an inherited syndrome that places members at increased risk for developing leukemia and other cancers. Eventually, genetic alteration should fulfill a vital need in the prevention and treatment of many diseases, including leukemia.

As discussed in chapters 2 and 8, the Philadelphia-chromosome translocation (1960) identified a subset among patients who had CML. Later investigators, however, using molecular techniques, recognized a new gene, the *bcr-abl* gene, in these patients. Subsequently, *bcr-abl* was demonstrated in the leukemia cells of some patients who were Ph[1] negative. The diagnosis of CML is now made definitively by establishing the presence of this hybrid gene, and the requisite probe for studying the gene is commercially available.

The *bcr-abl* gene has never been found in normal persons or in the normal somatic cells of patients who have CML. It apparently occurs uniquely in the leukemic cells of these patients and, therefore, must characterize the malignant clone. It represents a precise difference between the normal cell and the cancer cell. If the cancer cell can thus be distinguished at the molecular level, perhaps a method to eliminate the malignant clone will be forthcoming.

Cytogenetic and molecular techniques have revealed extensive multiformity in each leukemic disorder. These differences are becoming the basis for our enlightenment into the biology of leukemia because each abnormality is specific for the neoplasm. Cytogenetic and molecular investigations are now essential for diagnosis, staging, choice of therapy, early recognition of residual disease, and prognosis. As a result of these investigations, new directions in the diagnosis and therapy of leukemia are already being explored.

TEN

Future Directions

The future is the past again,
entered through another gate.

Sir Arthur Wing Pinero (1855–1934)

Before considering guidelines for future development, it is always helpful to look back, as we have done in this book, over the history of a field of endeavor for a chart or compass to pilot us. It is astonishing to recall that before 1946 there was essentially no specific treatment available for leukemia; along with a pessimistic prognosis patients received only blood transfusions or radiation. Today, therapies are available for all types of hematologic malignancies. Not all are curative, but most can offer extension of life with improved quality and, of prime importance, hope. Advances are occurring at a rapid rate, and it is not unrealistic for patients to anticipate and expect that better therapies for their disease will be imminently forthcoming. Present day treatment strategies have already diminished the hopelessness that accompanied the diagnosis of leukemia.

Unfortunately, only a small percentage of the worldwide population of patients with leukemia has access to frontline therapy. If absolute cures for all types of leukemia existed today, global mortality from leukemia would decrease by only a small percentage.[1]

STEM CELL

Sidney Farber referred to acute leukemia in children[2] and did not attempt to separate the disorder into various types according to the form it manifested.[1] Researchers are currently questioning the partition of leukemia into lymphocytic or myelocytic lineage, and it seems clear that a small percentage of patients have acute leukemia of complex origin and multilineage expression. Conversions or change-overs are also being reported. As described in chapter 8, a patient with Ph[1]-positive CML presenting in blast crisis may demonstrate totally the lymphoid phenotype, but when complete remission is achieved the karyotype remains essentially 100 percent Ph[1] positive—indicating derivation from a myeloid leukemic cell.

It is presently possible to grow myeloid stem cells in vitro; these generate platelets, red cells, granulocytes, and monocytes. Similarly, lymphoid stem cells create T-, B-, or null-cell forms. At some point in the embryologic evolution of a fetus, there is a cell that is mother to both the myeloid and lymphoid stem cells. Whether the mother cell still exists and maintains a role in the mature person is not known. Such a cell would have significance in bone marrow transplantation as both myeloid and lymphoid lines must be replaced and must be under correct guidance and control.

It seems apparent that leukemia and other cancers are genetic disorders. They are not analogous to congenital genetic diseases because they are not contained in the genome at birth. Rather, they are acquired changes that become well established in the genes of the affected cells. The characteristic features of the leukemia, such as its morphology, natural history, and response to various treatments, may be related to the genetic disarrangement and may not be indicative of lymphoid or myeloid lineage.[1]

A mutation, a permanent transmissible change in genetic material, may be inherited as a constitutional defect, but a gene must be mutated in both homologous chromosomes to convert a normal cell into a malignant one.[3,4] Therefore, a minimum of two changes is required. With the discovery of a human T cell leukemia virus, it became clear that a virus, as well as radiation or chemicals, can initiate a malignant mutation. In some unknown manner, mutations may confer a survival advantage on the clone, and it flourishes and thrives to the detriment of the normal cells, gradually becoming stronger and stronger as it invades and metastasizes.[5]

The regulation and control of the stem cell that is capable of malignant transformation would be a major breakthrough. Recognition and identification of the cell that is stem to the leukemic cell is likely to occur soon. Workers in the field of biologic response modifiers have already caught a glimpse of the likelihood of finding proteins that influence the transformation to malignancy and have the potential for regulating proliferation and differentiation. Other substances capable of inducing differentiation have already been reported, and this may become a realistic approach to therapy of the leukemias.

KARYOTYPIC CHANGES

It is certain that cytogenetic techniques will continue to improve and will become more available. Knowledge of nonrandom chromosomal patterns has revealed remarkable heterogeneity in leukemic disease, and the identification of specific subsets of patients has proven to be important for diagnosis, choice of treatment, and prognosis.

Methods will be developed for banding analysis of all 46 chromosomes, using a prompt, low-cost, practicable technique, and this will be included in the initial workup for each patient who has a leukemic disorder. The abnormal gene products that allow the detection of oncogenes also show promise for the discovery of minimal disease both in early detection and in discerning residual malignancy.

In the future, therapy that is toxic to normal cells will become obsolete, and treatment for a patient who has leukemia may consist of diagnosing a surplus, a shortage, or a disproportion in regulators and prescribing suitable measures to restore the necessary regulatory components consistent with a normal healthy individual. In other words, it should be possible to identify regulatory proteins that would counteract or prevent the transformation of a normal stem cell into a malignant stem cell that gives rise to all of the offspring making up a neoplasm.

Oncogenes and their protein products may be specific or definitive for cancer cells. They may be vital for the growth and proliferation of the tumor cell. Therefore, they may represent good targets for antineoplastic therapy that would be very precise and would not affect normal cells.[6]

Today it is just beginning to become apparent that there are multiple channels by which tumor progression could be modified. As a malignancy develops by stages, different types of genes and different processes come into play. The products of the stimulatory oncogenes may be involved in any step of the growth regulatory cycle, and suppressor genes may similarly extend over the entire scope of growth activities.[7]

In the 1980s the characteristic of malignant tumors to invade and metastasize occupied many prominent investigators. Various influential factors were reported, and, in some instances, specific genes and the mechanisms fundamental to their altered function were described. Such studies surely will be accomplished for other properties of malignant tumors that promote expansion, such as drug resistance, rapid growth rate, and deviations in antigenicity.[7]

As tumors evolve and progress, sequential genetic changes may occur. Tumor cells seem to be more unstable genetically than are normal cells. Sequential genetic changes have been documented extensively in CGL, and similar patterns occur frequently among these patients. Persons who have CLL, however, do not acquire additional karyotypic changes nearly as often, suggesting firmly established differences in the genetic permanence of the leukemic cells in the two disorders.[7]

Another exciting area for tomorrow's medicine will be the elucidation of the entire human genome, followed by synthesis of the complete gamut of gene products. This is predicting very far into the future, but, eventually, we may have access to regulatory proteins specific for the defect that is the result of a particular genetic mutation. We could then, for example, restore or prevent the transformation from a normal stem cell with diploid cytogenetics to a Ph^1-positive stem cell, which generates all of the offspring typifying chronic granulocytic leukemia.

BONE MARROW TRANSPLANTATION

Chapter 6 contained a discussion of a graft-versus-leukemia effect in allogeneic marrow recipients who have graft-versus-host disease. Studies have revealed a decreased rate of leukemia relapse in these persons when compared with recipients of syngeneic marrow or with allogeneic recipients who do not have graft-versus-host disease. Graft-versus-host disease seems to enhance the opportunity for disease-free survival. Evidence of an involved interrelation between the recipient's bone marrow stromal cells and the donor's myeloid stem cells has been reported; descriptions of a lymphoid-myeloid interplay contribute added confusion. Therapy that inhibits or destroys lymphoid cells in the recipient is being investigated.

At present, we know enough about the immunologic changes occurring in posttransplant patients to realize that we have only a rudimentary acquaintance with the subject. Major advances of our knowledge in this area seem to be on the threshold and will inevitably have a significant effect on transplantation.

Autologous Bone Marrow Transplantation

Today, bone marrow cells can be collected from a patient when there is no evidence of disease, as in first remission, preserved for long periods, and infused back into the person whenever needed. It requires about 2 to 3 weeks for these cells to reconstitute the bone marrow after total-body irradiation. Granulocyte-macrophage colony-stimulating factor, however, reduces the period of neutropenia after autologous marrow transplantation from 16 to 10 days.[8]

Bone marrow can be treated in the laboratory with drugs or with monoclonal antibodies in an attempt to eradicate residual leukemic cells as long as the substance used is not severely toxic to hematopoietic stem cells and can be eliminated or diluted to nontoxic levels before the marrow is returned to the patient.

In the future, with the availability of the required stimulators and regulators, it should be possible to provoke some of the autologous stem cells to finish their cycle of differentiation in vitro so that mature granulocytes, platelets, and erythrocytes would be on hand to replenish the bone marrow. There would be no 3-week waiting period; the patient would be protected from the cytopenias that follow bone marrow damage.

Autologous bone marrow will become a very active and intense field for investigational work that may eventually affect many facets of cancer treatment.

COLONY-STIMULATING FACTORS

Differentiation of bone marrow cells seems to be prompted by determinate hematopoietic growth factors. The colony-stimulating factors (CSFs), described briefly in chapter 7, may provide the required impetus for maturation of these cells.

The genes for macrophage (M) and granulocyte-macrophage (GM) CSFs and for M-CSF receptor and those for interleukins 3, 4, and 5 are all clustered on chromosome 5.[9-11] It has been suggested that one or more of these may be involved in a clinical syndrome called 5q−, in which there is a deletion of the long arm of chromosome 5. This was described in chapter 8 in regard to patients with ANLL who had previously been treated for a different malignancy or who had been exposed to radiation or cytotoxic agents.

A translocation between chromosomes 15 and 17 occurs in promyelocytic leukemia, and the granulocyte (G) CSF gene normally resides on number 17. Therefore, the lack of the differentiation stimulus usually supplied by this gene may cause a maturation block at the promyelocyte stage.[9,12]

In all cases of AML there seems to be a block to the normal maturation of blast cells.[9] Do the CSFs play a role in the genesis or continuance of the myeloid leukemias? Would the treatment of patients who have these leukemias be enhanced by modifying the amounts or proportions of one or more of the CSFs?[9]

In vitro studies indicate that at the time of diagnosis most myeloid leukemias require exogenous CSF to proliferate, although there are a few that do not. Many leukemias in blast crisis do not proliferate in vitro even in the presence of CSF.[9] Perhaps some growth factor, still to be described, is stimulating their proliferation in vivo. Morstyn, Burgess, Metcalf, and colleagues, separately and jointly, have explored and written extensively on the hematopoietic growth factors. Their work, as well as that of many others, has contributed to an extensive and rapidly growing compilation of knowledge about these factors and their functions. The activities of the growth factors are very specific, and expectations are high that their use will initiate innovative therapeutic approaches, not only in transplantation and the leukemias but also for solid tumors.

A CURE FOR CANCER?

Many cytogeneticists have expressed surprise at the frequency with which they encounter mutations. Genetic alterations are not at all unusual and are seen more often in older persons. In living organisms, cells must constantly be replaced and restored; thus, exact duplicates of individual cells must be produced, and stem cells must be regulated and guided through the complicated steps of differentiation into specialized cells to form tissues and organs. These processes are fraught with the constant danger of errors. Constitutional fragility syndromes, as well as exposure to viruses, radiation, and chemicals, can increase the potential for mutations, and humans have never been able to protect themselves totally from such influences. Even if this were possible, deviations seem to be inevitable.

Today, with people living longer lives, cumulative alterations in genes, as well as loss of suppressor gene functions through combinations of inherited and somatic deletions or other mechanisms,[7] seem more probable. As life-span increases, the risk of malignancy becomes higher, and certain cytogenetic aberrations seen in older persons are rarely encountered in the young.

Therefore, it is doubtful that we will ever be successful in eradicating or eliminating cancer as a disease; we probably will not be able to prevent it. We hope and anticipate that we will learn to detect it at a very early stage and that we will acquire the knowledge and means to provide prolonged control to all patients, not just a privileged few.

References

Preface

1. Sandberg A: Editorial. *Cancer Genet Cytogenet* 28:1, 1987
2. Cook D: Meet the archbishop of controversy. *Look Magazine*, pp. 85–89, March 17, 1959
3. Pollock MR: The discovery of DNA: An ironic tale of chance, prejudice and insight. *J Gen Microbiol* 63:1–20, 1970

1. Before the Twentieth Century

1. Velpeau A: *Rev Med* 2:218, 1827. Quoted by Virchow: *Med Z* 16:9, 15, 1847
2. Dameshek W, Gunz F: *Leukemia*, ed. 2. New York, Grune & Stratton, pp. 1–11, 1964
3. Lehndorff H: Leukemia one hundred years ago. *Arch Pediatr* 72:26–30, 1955
4. Dreyfus C: *Some Milestones in the History of Hematology*. New York, Grune & Stratton, pp. 54–62, 1957
5. Donné A: *Cours de Microscopie*. Paris, Baillière, pp. 10–12, 1844
6. Thorburn AL: Alfred Francois Donné, 1801–1878, discoverer of *Trichomonas vaginalis* and of leukemia. *Br J Venereal Dis* 50:377–380, 1974
7. Bennett JH: *On the Employment of the Microscope in Medical Studies*. Edinburgh, M. Stewart & Co., 1841
8. Bennett JH: Hypertrophy of the spleen and liver, in which death took place from suppuration of the blood. *Edinburgh Med Surg J* 64:413–423, 1845
9. Virchow R: Weisses Blut. *Neue Notizen Gebiete Natur-Heilkunde* 36:151–157, 1845
10. Seufert W, Seufert WD: The recognition of leukemia as a systemic disease. *J Hist Med Allied Sci* 37:34–50, 1982
11. Virchow R: Zur pathologischen Physiologie des Bluts: II. Weisses Blut (Leukämie). *Virchows Arch Pathol Anat Physiol* 1:563–572, 1847

12. Virchow R: Zur pathologischen Physiologie des Bluts: IV. Farblose, pigmentirte und geschwänzte, nicht specifische Zellen im Blut. *Virchows Arch Pathol Anat Physiol* 2:587–598, 1849

13. Virchow R: Über farblose Blutkörperchern und Leukämie. In *Gesammelte Abhandlungen zur wissenschaftlichen Medizin.* Frankfurt, Verlag von Meidlinger Sohn, pp. 147–153, 1856

14. Virchow R: Zur pathologischen Physiologie des Bluts: Die Bedeutung der Milz- und Lymphdrüsen-Krankheiten für die Blutmischung (Leukaemie). *Virchows Arch Pathol Anat Physiol* 5:43–128, 1853

15. Schoenberg DG, Schoenberg BS: Eponym: Nikolaus Friedreich and ataxia: Tabes or not tabes? *South Med J* 70:749, 1977

16. Friedreich N: Ein neuer Fall von Leukämie. *Virchows Arch Pathol Anat Physiol* 12:37–68, 1857

17. Cahen: Discussion. *Bull Soc Med Hop* 3:55, 1856

18. Barthez F: Discussion. *Bull Soc Med Hop* 3:55, 1856

19. Schoenberg BS: Joseph Janvier Woodward and an early American view of cancer. *Surg Gynecol Obstet* 136:456–462, 1973

20. Woodward JJ: On the use of aniline in histological researches: With a method of investigating the histology of the human intestine, and remarks on some of the points to be observed in the study of the diseased intestine in camp fevers and diarrhoeas. *Am J Med Sci* 49:106–113, 1865

21. Neumann E: Ein Fall von Leukämie mit Erkrankung des Knochenmarkes. *Arch Heilk* 11:1–15, 1870

22. Neumann E: Farblose Blut- und Eiterzellen. *Klin Wochenschr* 15:607–608, 1878

23. Rauscher FJ Jr, Shimkin MB: Viral oncology. In *NIH: An Account of Research in Its Laboratories and Clinics*, Stettem D Jr, Carrigan WT (eds.). Orlando, FL, Academic Press, pp. 350–367, 1984

24. Gowers WR: Splenic leucocythaemia. In *A System of Medicine*, vol. 3, Reynolds JR (ed.). Philadelphia, H.C. Lea's Son & Co., pp. 476–528, 1880

25. Ehrlich P: *Farbenanalytische Untersuchungen zur Histologie und Klinik des Bluts.* Berlin, A. Hirschwald, 1891

26. Rosenthal N: The lymphomas and leukemias. *Bull NY Acad Med* 30:583–600, 1954

27. Pelner L: A warm portrait of Paul Ehrlich. *Med Times* 99(12):110–120, 1971

28. Bennett JM: Myelomonocytic leukemias: A historical review and perspectives. *Cancer* 27:1218–1220, 1971

29. Naegeli O: Über rothes Knochenmark und Myeloblasten. *Dtsch Med Wochenschr* 26:287–290, 1900

30. Auer J: Some hitherto undescribed structures in the large lymphocytes in a case of acute leukemia. *Am J Med Sci* 131:1002–1015, 1906

31. Reschad H, Schilling-Torgau V: Über eine neue Leukämie durch echte Übergangsformen (Splenozytenleukämie) und ihre Bedeutung für die Selbstständigkeit dieser Zellen. *Munchen Med Wochenschr* 60:1981–1984, 1913

2. Etiology

1. Furth J, Kahn MC: The transmission of leukemia of mice with a single cell. *Am J Cancer* 31:276–282, 1937
2. Yarbro JW: The new biology of cancer: Future clinical applications. *Semin Oncol* 16:254–259, 1989
3. Borrel A: Epithélioses infectieuses et epithéliomas. *Ann Inst Pasteur* 17:81–122, 1903
4. Wintrobe MM: *Clinical Hematology*, ed. 8. Philadelphia, Lea & Febiger, pp. 1449–1492, 1981
5. Ellermann V, Bang O: Experimentelle Leukämie bei Hühnern. *Zentralbl Bakteriol Parasitenkunde Infektionskrankheiten 1. Abt Orig* 46:595–609, 1908
6. Gross L: Viral etiology of leukemia and lymphomas in mice: A brief historical survey and present status. *Zentralbl Bakteriol Parasitenkunde Infektion Hyg 1. Abt Orig Reihe A* 220:57–65, 1972
7. Gross L: "Spontaneous" leukemia developing in C3H mice following inoculation, in infancy, with Ak-leukemic extracts, or Ak-embryos. *Proc Soc Exp Biol* 76:27–32, 1951
8. Negroni G: Isolation of viruses from leukaemic patients. *Br Med J* 1:927–929, 1964
9. Nowell PC: Phytohemagglutinin induces DNA synthesis in leucocyte cultures. *Cancer Res* 20:462–471, 1960
10. Gallo RC: Human T-cell leukaemia/lymphoma virus and T-cell malignancies in adults. In *Cancer Surveys*, vol. 3, Wyke J, Weiss R (eds.). Oxford, Oxford University Press, pp. 113–159, 1984
11. Morgan DA, Ruscetti FW, Gallo RC: Selective in vitro growth of T-lymphocytes from normal human bone marrow. *Science* 193:1007–1008, 1976
12. Poiesz BJ, Ruscetti FW, Gazdar AF, et al: Detection and isolation of type C retrovirus particles from fresh and cultured lymphocytes of a patient with cutaneous T-cell lymphoma. *Proc Natl Acad Sci USA* 77:7415–7419, 1980
13. Poiesz BJ, Ruscetti FW, Mier JW, et al: T-cell lines established from human T-lymphocytic neoplasias by direct response to T-cell growth factor. *Proc Natl Acad Sci USA* 77:6815–6819, 1980
14. Kalyanaraman VS, Sarngadharan MG, Robert-Guroff M, et al: A new subtype of human T-cell leukemia virus (HTLV-II) associated with a variant of hairy cell leukemia. *Science* 218:571–573, 1982
15. Barre-Sinoussi F, Chermann JC, Rey F, et al: Isolation of a T-lymphotropic retrovirus from a patient at risk for acquired immunodeficiency syndrome (AIDS). *Science* 220:868–871, 1983
16. Popovic M, Sarngadharan MG, Read E, et al: Detection, isolation, and continuous production of cytopathic retroviruses (HTLV-III) from patients with AIDS and pre-AIDS. *Science* 224:497–500, 1984
17. Gallo RC, Salahuddin SZ, Popovic M, et al: Frequent detection and iso-

lation of cytopathic retroviruses (HTLV-III) from patients with AIDS and at risk for AIDS. *Science* 224:500–503, 1984

18. Levy JA, Hoffman AD, Kramer SM, et al: Isolation of lymphocytopathic retroviruses from San Francisco patients with AIDS. *Science* 225:840–842, 1984

19. Wong R: AIDS update: History, disease manifestations, and transmission. *Am Pharm* NS27(8):28–33, 1987

20. Ratner L, Haseltine W, Patarca R, et al: Complete nucleotide sequence of the AIDS virus, HTLV-III. *Nature* 313:277–283, 1985

21. Hahn BH, Shaw GM, Taylor ME, et al: Genetic variation in HTLV-III/LAV over time in patients with AIDS or at risk for AIDS. *Science* 232:1548–1553, 1986

22. Siliciano RF, Lawton T, Knall C, et al: Analysis of host-virus interactions in AIDS with anti-gp120 T cell clones: Effect of HIV sequence variation and a mechanism for CD4$^+$ cell depletion. *Cell* 54:561–575, 1988

23. Shaw GM, Broder S, Essex M, et al: Human T-cell leukemia virus: Its discovery and role in leukemogenesis and immunosuppression. *Adv Intern Med* 30:1–27, 1984

24. von Jagié N, Schwarz G, von Siebenrock L: Blutbefunde bei Röntgenologen. *Klin Wochenschr* 48:120, 1911

25. March HC: Leukemia in radiologists. *Radiology* 43:275–278, 1944

26. Cronkite EP: Evidence for radiation and chemicals as leukemogenic agents. *Arch Environ Health* 3:297–303, 1961

27. Misao T, Haraguchi Y, Hattori K: A case of monocytic leukemia developed after the acute symptoms by atomic bomb exposure. In *Collection of the Reports on the Investigation of the Atomic Bomb Casualties*, vol. 2, Science Council of Japan (ed.). Tokyo, Nihon Gakujutsu Shinkōkai, 1953 (in Japanese)

28. Committee for the Compilation of Materials on Damage Caused by the Atomic Bombs in Hiroshima and Nagasaki: *The Physical, Medical, and Social Effects of the Atomic Bombings*, translated from Japanese by Ishikawa E and Swain DL. New York, Basic Books, pp. 255–276, 1981

29. Komiya E, Yamamoto S: A case of acute leukemia of survivors of the atomic bomb. *Shindan to Chiryō (Diagnosis and Treatment)* 35:88, 1947

30. Ichimaru M, Ishimaru T: Review of thirty years' study of Hiroshima and Nagasaki atomic bomb survivors: II. Biological effects. D: Leukemia and related disorders. *J Radiat Res (Tokyo)*, 16(Suppl):89–96, 1975

31. Chen E: Low-dose radiation riskier than believed. *Houston Chronicle*, p. 2A, December 20, 1989

32. Gunz FW: The epidemiology and genetics of the chronic leukemias. *Clin Hematol* 6:3–20, 1977

33. Court-Brown WM, Doll R: Mortality from cancer and other causes after radiotherapy for ankylosing spondylitis. *Br Med J* 2:1327–1332, 1965

34. Shimkin MB, Triolo VA: History of chemical carcinogenesis: Some prospective remarks. *Prog Exp Tumor Res* 11:1–20, 1969

35. Pott P: *Chirurgical Observations Relative to the Cataract, the Polypus of the Nose, the Cancer of the Scrotum, the different kinds of ruptures,*

and the mortification of the toes and feet. London, Hawes, Clarke, & Collins, 1775

36. Bett WR: Historical aspects of cancer. In *Cancer*, vol. 1, Raven RW (ed.). London, Butterworth & Co., pp. 1–5, 1957

37. Klein E, Schwartz RA: Cancer and the skin. In *Cancer Medicine*, Holland JF, Frei E III (eds.). Philadelphia, Lea & Febiger, pp. 2057–2108, 1982

38. Selling L: Preliminary report of some cases of purpura haemorrhagica due to benzol poisoning. *Bull Johns Hopkins Hosp* 21:33–37, 1910

39. Dameshek W: Control of leukemia. *N Engl J Med* 250:131–139, 1954

40. Delore P, Borgomano C: Leucémie aigue au cours de l'intoxication benzènique: Sur l'origine toxique de certaines leucémies aigues et leurs relation avec les anémies graves. *J Med Lyon* 9:227–233, 1928

41. Lignac GOE: Die Benzolleukämie bei Menschen und weissen Mäusen. *Krankheitsforschung* 9:403–453, 1932

42. Morton JJ, Mider GB: The production of lymphomatosis in mice of known genetic constitution. *Science* 87:327–328, 1938

43. Latta JS, Davies LT: Effects on the blood and hemopoietic organs of the albino rat of repeated administration of benzene. *Arch Pathol* 31:55–67, 1941

44. Forni A, Moreo L: Cytogenetic studies in a case of benzene leukemia. *Eur J Cancer* 3:251–255, 1967

45. Dean BJ: Genetic toxicology of benzene, toluene, xylenes and phenols. *Mutat Res* 47:75–97, 1978

46. Sandberg AA: *Chromosomes in Human Cancer and Leukemia.* New York, Elsevier North Holland, pp. 441–442, 1980

47. Videbaek A: *Heredity in Human Leukemia and its Relation to Cancer.* Copenhagen, Arnold Busck, 1947

48. Kolmeier KH, Bayrd EO: Familial leukemia: Report of instance and review of the literature. *Proc Mayo Clin* 38:523–531, 1963

49. Harnden DG: Inherited factors in leukaemia and lymphoma. *Leuk Res* 9:705–707, 1985

50. Nowell PC: Chromosomal and molecular clues to tumor progression. *Semin Oncol* 16:116–127, 1989

51. Brewster HF, Cannon HE: Acute lymphatic leukemia: A report of a case in 11th month mongolian idiot. *New Orleans Med Surg J* 82:872–873, 1930

52. Stewart A, Webb J, Hewitt D: A survey of childhood malignancies. *Br Med J* 1:1495–1508, 1958

53. Boveri T: Über mehrpolige Mitosen als Mittel zur Analyse des Zellkerns. *Verh Physikal Med Ges* 35:67–88, 1902

54. Whang-Peng J, Knutsen T: The role of cytogenetics in the characterization of acute leukemia: Acute lymphoblastic leukemia and acute myeloblastic leukemia. In *The Acute Leukemias: Biologic, Diagnostic, and Therapeutic Determinants*, Stass SA (ed.). New York, Marcel Dekker, pp. 153–201, 1987

55. Nowell PC, Hungerford DA: Chromosome studies on normal and leukemic human leukocytes. *JNCI* 25:85–109, 1960

56. Osgood EE, Krippaehne ML: The gradient tissue culture method. *Exp Cell Res* 9:116–127, 1955

57. Tjio JH, Levan A: The chromosome number of man. *Hereditas* 42:1–6, 1956

58. Nowell PC: This week's citation classic. *Current Contents* 8:19, February 25, 1985

59. Nowell PC, Hungerford DA: A minute chromosome in human chronic granulocytic leukemia (abstract). *Science* 132:1497, 1960

60. Baikie AG, Court-Brown WM, Buckton KE, et al: A possible specific chromosome abnormality in human chronic myeloid leukaemia. *Nature* 188:1165–1166, 1960

61. Tough IM, Court-Brown WM, Baikie AG, et al: Cytogenetic studies in chronic myeloid leukaemia and acute leukaemia associated with mongolism. *Lancet* 1:411–417, 1961

62. Nowell PC, Hungerford DA: Chromosome studies in human leukemia: II. Chronic granulocytic leukemia. *JNCI* 27:1013–1021, 1961

63. Sandberg AA, Ishihara T, Miwa T, et al: The in vivo constitution of marrow from 34 human leukemias and 60 nonleukemic controls. *Cancer Res* 21:678–689, 1961

64. Whang-Peng J, Knutsen T: Chromosomal abnormalities. In *Chronic Granulocytic Leukaemia*, Shaw MT (ed.). New York, Praeger, pp. 49–92, 1982

65. Prieto F, Egozcue J, Forteza G, et al: Identification of the Philadelphia (Ph¹) chromosome. *Blood* 35:23–28, 1970

66. Caspersson T, Gahrton G, Lindsten J, et al: Identification of the Philadelphia chromosome as number 22 by quinacrine mustard fluorescence. *Exp Cell Res* 63:238–244, 1970

67. Rowley JD: A new consistent abnormality in chronic myelogenous leukemia identified by quinacrine fluorescence and Giemsa staining. *Nature* 243:290–293, 1973

68. Lawler SD: The cytogenetics of chronic granulocytic leukemia. *Clin Hematol* 6:55–75, 1977

69. Ezdinli EZ, Sokal JE, Crosswhite L, et al: Philadelphia-chromosome-positive and -negative chronic myelocytic leukemia. *Ann Intern Med* 72:175–182, 1970

70. Canellos GP: The treatment of chronic granulocytic leukemia. *Clin Hematol* 6:113–128, 1977

71. Freireich EJ: Hematologic malignancies: Adult acute leukemia. *Hosp Pract* 21:91–110, 1986

72. Dewald GW, Noel P, Dahl RJ, et al: Chromosome abnormalities in malignant hematologic disorders. *Proc Mayo Clin* 60:675–689, 1985

73. Stich HF: Chromosomes of tumor cells: I. Murine leukemias induced by one or two injections of 7,12-dimethylbenz[α] anthracene. *JNCI* 25:649–661, 1960

74. Dofuku R, Biedler JL, Spengler BH, et al: Trisomy of chromosome 15 in spontaneous leukemia of AKR mice. *Proc Natl Acad Sci USA* 72:1515–1517, 1975

75. Nordling CO: A new theory on the cancer-inducing mechanism. *Br J Cancer* 7:68–72, 1953
76. Ashley DJB: The two "hit" and multiple "hit" theories of carcinogenesis. *Br J Cancer* 23:313–328, 1969
77. Knudson AG Jr: Mutation and cancer: Statistical study of retinoblastoma. *Proc Natl Acad Sci USA* 68:820–823, 1971
78. Hsu T-C: Genetic predisposition to cancer with special reference to mutagen sensitivity. *In Vitro Cell Dev Biol* 23:591–603, 1987
79. SoRelle R: Genetics offers some cancer answers. *Houston Chronicle*, p. 7B, August 1, 1988
80. Collins SJ, Kubonishi I, Miyoshi I, et al: Altered transcription of the c-*abl* oncogene in K–562 and other chronic myelogenous leukemia cells. *Science* 225:72–74, 1984
81. Canaani E, Steiner-Saltz D, Aghai E, et al: Altered transcription of an oncogene in chronic myeloid leukaemia. *Lancet* 1:593–595, 1984
82. de Klein A, van Kessel AG, Grosveld G, et al: A cellular oncogene is translocated to the Philadelphia chromosome in chronic myelocytic leukemia. *Nature* 300:765–767, 1982
83. Heisterkamp N, Groffen J, Stephenson J, et al: Chromosomal localization of human cellular homologues of two viral oncogenes. *Nature* 299:747–749, 1982
84. Dalla Favera R, Gallo R, Giallongo A, et al: Chromosomal localization of the human homolog (c-*sis*) of the simian sarcoma virus *onc* gene. *Science* 218:686–688, 1982
85. Kloetzer W, Kurzrock R, Smith L, et al: The human cellular *abl* gene product in the chronic myelogenous leukemia cell line K562 has an associated tyrosine protein kinase activity. *Virology* 140:230–238, 1985
86. Ben-Neriah Y, Daley GQ, Mes-Masson A-M, et al: The chronic myelogenous leukemia-specific P210 protein is the product of the *bcr/abl* hybrid gene. *Science* 233:212–214, 1986
87. Konopka JB, Watanabe SM, Witte ON: An alteration of the human c-*abl* protein in K562 leukemia cells unmasks associated tyrosine kinase activity. *Cell* 37:1035–1042, 1984
88. Konopka JB, Watanabe SM, Singer JW, et al: Cell lines and clinical isolates derived from Ph¹-positive chronic myelogenous leukemia patients express c-*abl* proteins with a common structural alteration. *Proc Natl Acad Sci USA* 82:1810–1814, 1985
89. Maxwell SA, Kurzrock R, Parsons SJ, et al: Analysis of P210 *bcr abl* tyrosine protein kinase activity in various subtypes of Philadelphia chromosome-positive cells from chronic myelogenous leukemia patients. *Cancer Res* 47:1731–1739, 1987
90. Kantarjian HM, Keating MJ, Walters RS, et al: Clinical and prognostic features of Philadelphia chromosome-negative chronic myelogenous leukemia. *Cancer* 58:2023–2030, 1986
91. Kantarjian HM, Shtalrid M, Kurzrock R, et al: Significance and correlations of molecular analysis results in patients with Philadelphia chro-

mosome-negative chronic myelogenous leukemia and chronic myelomonocytic leukemia. *Am J Med* 85:639–644, 1988

92. Adler KR, Lempert N, Scharfman WB: Chronic granulocytic leukemia
following successful renal transplantation. *Cancer* 41:2206–2208, 1978

93. Lubynski R, Meyers AM, Disler PB: Chronic granulocytic leukemia in
a patient with a renal allograft. *Arch Intern Med* 138:1429–1430, 1978

94. Mooy JMV, Hagenouw-Taal JCW, Lameijer LDF: Chronic granulocytic
leukemia in a renal transplant recipient. *Cancer* 41:7–9, 1978

95. Frei E III: Summary and perspectives. In *Hodgkin's Disease and Non-
Hodgkin's Lymphoma: New Perspectives in Immunotherapy, Diagnosis,
and Treatment. University of Texas M. D. Anderson Clinical Conference
on Cancer*, vol. 27, Ford RJ Jr, Fuller LM, Hagemeister FB (eds.). New
York, Raven Press, pp. 427–434, 1983

96. Kingston JE, Hawkins MM, Draper GJ, et al: Patterns of multiple primary
tumours in patients treated for cancer during childhood. *Br J Cancer*
56:331–338, 1987

3. Early Research in Cancer Chemotherapy at the National Cancer Institute

1. Sessions SM: Review of the Cancer Chemotherapy National Service Center Program: Development and organization. *Cancer Chemother Rep* 7:25–
64, 1960

2. DeVita VT Jr: On special initiatives, critics, and the National Cancer
Program. *Cancer Treat Rep* 68:1–4, 1984

3. Zubrod CG: Historic milestones in curative chemotherapy. *Semin Oncol*
6:490–505, 1979

4. Zubrod CG: Origins and development of chemotherapy research at the
National Cancer Institute. *Cancer Treat Rep* 68:9–19, 1984

5. DeVita VT Jr: Quoted in *Cancer Lett* 5(2):March 23, 1979

6. Shorter E: *The Health Century*. New York, Doubleday, pp. 179–211, 1987

7. Schmidt BC: Five years into the National Cancer Program: Retrospective
perspectives—the National Cancer Act of 1971. *JNCI* 59:687–692, 1977

8. Goldin A, Mantel N, Greenhouse SW, et al: Factors influencing the specificity of action of an antileukemic agent (aminopterin): Time of treatment and dosage schedule. *Cancer Res* 14:311–314, 1954

9. Goldin A, Venditti JM, Humphreys SR, et al: A quantitative comparison
of the antileukemic effectiveness of two folic acid antagonists. *JNCI*
15:1657–1664, 1955

10. Goldin A, Venditti JM, Humphreys SR, et al: Modification of treatment
schedules in the management of advanced mouse leukemia with amethopterin. *JNCI* 17:203–212, 1956

11. Goldin A, Venditti JM, Humphreys SR, et al: Factors influencing the
specificity of action of an antileukemic agent (aminopterin): Host age
and weight. *JNCI* 16:709–721, 1955

12. Goldin A, Venditti JM, Humphreys SR, et al: Influence of the concentration of leukemic inoculum on the effectiveness of treatment. *Science*
123:840, 1956

13. Lane M: Chemotherapy of cancer. In *Cancer*, ed. 5, del Regato JA, Spjut HJ (eds.). St. Louis, C.V. Mosby, pp. 105–130, 1977
14. Sauberlich HE, Baumann CA: A factor required for the growth of *Leuconostoc citrovorum*. *J Biol Chem* 176:165–173, 1948
15. Goldin A, Mantel N, Greenhouse SW, et al: Estimation of the antileukemic potency of the antimetabolite aminopterin, administration alone and in combination with citrovorum factor or folic acid. *Cancer Res* 13:843–850, 1953
16. Goldin A, Venditti JM, Humphreys SR, et al: Factors influencing the specificity of action of an antileukemic agent (aminopterin): Multiple treatment schedules plus delayed administration of citrovorum factor. *Cancer Res* 15:57–61, 1955
17. Goldin A, Serpick AA, Mantel N: Experimental screening procedures and clinical predictability value. *Cancer Chemother Rep* 50:173–218, 1966
18. Goldin A, Carter S, Mantel N: Evaluation of antineoplastic activity: Requirements of test systems. In *Antineoplastic and Immunosuppressive Agents*, vol. 1, Sartorelli AC, Johns DG (eds.). Berlin, Springer-Verlag, pp. 12–32, 1974
19. Law LW, Dunn TB, Boyle PJ, et al: Observations on the effect of a folic-acid antagonist on transplantable lymphoid leukemias in mice. *JNCI* 10:179–192, 1949
20. Law LW: Differences between cancers in terms of evolution of drug resistance. *Cancer Res* 16:698–716, 1956
21. Holland JF, Danielson E, Sahagian-Edwards A: Use of ethylene diamine tetra acetic acid in hypercalcemic patients. *Proc Soc Exp Biol Med* 84:359–364, 1953
22. Holland JF, Hosley H, Scharlau C, et al: A controlled trial of urethane treatment in multiple myeloma. *Blood* 27:328–342, 1966
23. Holland JF: Symposium on the Experimental Pharmacology and Clinical Use of Antimetabolites. Part VIII. Folic acid antagonists. *Clin Pharmacol Ther* 2:374–409, 1961
24. Holland JF, Scharlau C, Gailani S, et al: Vincristine treatment of advanced cancer: A cooperative study of 92 cases. *Cancer Res* 33:1258–1264, 1973
25. Holland JF: Breaking the cure barrier. *J Clin Oncol* 1:75–90, 1983
26. Holland JF: Randomized trials in rare tumors. *J Clin Oncol* 3:1163–1165, 1985
27. Holland JF: Adjuvant chemotherapy of osteosarcoma: No runs, no hits, two men left on base. *J Clin Oncol* 5:4–6, 1987

4. Chemotherapy with Single Agents

1. Zubrod CG: Historic milestones in curative chemotherapy. *Semin Oncol* 6:490–505, 1979
2. Creasey WA: Antineoplastic and immunosuppressive agents. In *Handbook of Experimental Pharmacology*, vol. 38 (ed. 2), Sartorelli AC, Johns DG (eds.). Berlin, Springer-Verlag, pp. 670–694, 1975
3. Farber S: Approaches to the chemotherapy of cancer. *Trans Stud Coll Physicians Phila* 23:74–82, 1955

4. Bett WR: Historical aspects of cancer. In *Cancer*, vol. 1, Raven RW (ed.). London, Butterworth, pp. 1–5, 1957

5. Lissauer H: Zwei Fälle von Leucaemie. *Klin Wochensch* 2:403, 1865

6. Beatson TG: On the treatment of inoperable cases of cancer of the mamma: Suggestions for a new method of treatment, with illustrative cases. *Lancet* 2:104–107, 162–165, 1896

7. Marshall EK Jr: Historical perspectives in chemotherapy. In *Advances in Chemotherapy*, Goldin A, Hawking F (eds.). New York, Academic Press, pp. 1–8, 1964

8. Ehrlich P: Über die Beziehungen von chemischer Constitution, Vertheilung und pharmakologischer Wirkung. Address before Verein für innere Medizen, 1898. In *The Collected Papers of Paul Ehrlich*, Himmelweit F (ed.). London, Pergamon, pp. 596–618, 1956

9. Hill DL: *A Review of Cyclophosphamide*. Springfield, IL, Charles C Thomas, p. 5, 1974

10. Haddow A: Summary and conclusions following presentations of papers on alkylating substances at the International Symposium on Chemotherapy of Cancer, Lugano, 1964. In *Chemotherapy of Cancer*, Plattner PA (ed.). Amsterdam, Elsevier, p. 73, 1964

11. Pusey WA: Report of cases treated with roentgen rays. *JAMA* 38:911–919, 1902

12. Goldman JM: The treatment of chronic granulocytic leukemia. In *Chronic Granulocytic Leukemia*, Shaw MT (ed.). New York, Praeger, pp. 189–216, 1982

13. Gunz FW: Chronic lymphocytic leukemia. In *Cancer Medicine*, Holland JF, Frei E III (eds.). Philadelphia, Lea & Febiger, pp. 1460–1477, 1982

14. Osler W: *Principles and Practice of Medicine*, ed. 7. New York, D. Appleton, p. 738, 1909

15. Shimkin MB: As memory serves: An informal history of the National Cancer Institute, 1937–57. *JNCI* 59(Suppl 2):559–600, 1977

16. Woglom WH: General review of cancer therapy. In *Approaches to Tumor Chemotherapy*, Moulton FR (ed.). Washington, DC, American Association for the Advancement of Science, pp. 1–10, 1947

17. Woglom WH: Immunity to transplantable tumors. *Cancer Rev* 4:129–195, 1929

18. Krumbhaar E, Krumbhaar H: The blood and bone marrow in yellow cross gas (mustard gas) poisoning. *J Med Res* 40:497–506, 1919

19. Meyer V: *Chemische Berichte (Weinheim)* 20:1725, 1887

20. Alexander SF: Medical report of the Bari Harbor mustard casualties. *Milit Surg* 101:1–17, 1947

21. Zubrod CG: The cure of cancer by chemotherapy: Reflections on how it happened. *Med Pediatr Oncol* 8:107–114, 1980

22. Gilman A: The initial clinical trial of nitrogen mustard. *Am J Surg* 105:574–578, 1963

23. Goodman LS, Wintrobe MM, Dameshek W, et al: Nitrogen mustard therapy. *JAMA* 132:126–132, 1946

24. Jacobson LO, Spurr CL, Barron ESG, et al: Nitrogen mustard therapy: Studies on the effect of methyl-bis (beta-chloroethyl) amine hydrochlo-

ride on neoplastic diseases and allied disorders of the hemopoietic system. *JAMA* 132:263–271, 1946

25. Karnofsky DA, Craver LF, Rhoads CP, et al: Evaluation of nitrogen mustards in the treatment of lymphomas, leukemia and allied diseases. In *Approaches to Tumor Chemotherapy*, Moulton FR (ed.). Washington, DC, American Association for the Advancement of Science, pp. 319 337, 1947

26. Heller JR: Cancer chemotherapy, history and present status. *Bull NY Acad Med* 38:348–363, 1962

27. Haddow A, Kon GAR, Ross WCJ: Effects upon tumours of various haloalkylarylamines. *Nature* 162:824–825, 1948

28. Haddow A, Timmis GM: Myleran in chronic myeloid leukemia. *Lancet* 1:207–208, 1953

29. Galton DAG: Myleran in chronic myeloid leukemia. *Lancet* 1:208–213, 1953

30. Tartaglia AP: Adult leukemia and the myeloproliferative disorders. In *Clinical Oncology*, Horton J, Hill GJ (eds.). Philadelphia, W.B. Saunders, pp. 727–746, 1977

31. Galton DAG, Israels LG, Nabarro JDN, et al: Clinical trials of p-(DI-2-chloroethylamino)-phenylbutyric acid (CB 1348) in malignant lymphoma. *Br Med J* 2:1172–1176, 1955

32. Arnold H, Bourseaux F, Brock N: Neuartige Krebs-Chemotherapeutica aus der Gruppe der zyklischen N-Lost-Phosphamidester. *Naturwissenschaften* 45:64–66, 1958

33. Brock N: Zur pharmakologischen Charakterisierung zyklischen N-Lost-Phosphamidester als Krebs-Chemotherapeutica. *Arzneimittelforschung* 8:1–9, 1958

34. Gross R: First experiments with Endoxan (B–518). Presented at Symposium: Chemotherapy of Malignant Tumors. Scientific Division, Asta-Werke A.G., Brockwede, Germany, December 18, 1957

35. Brock N, Hohorst HJ: Metabolism of cyclophosphamide. *Cancer* 20:900–904, 1967

36. Coggins PR, Ravdin RG, Eisman SH: Clinical pharmacology and preliminary evaluation of Cytoxan (cyclophosphamide). *Cancer Chemother Rep* 3:9–11, 1959

37. Foye LV Jr, Chapman CG, Willett FM, et al: Cyclophosphamide: A preliminary study of a new alkylating agent. *Cancer Chemother Rep* 6:39–40, 1960

38. Haar H, Marshall J, Bierman HR, et al: The influence of cyclophosphamide upon neoplastic diseases in man. *Cancer Chemother Rep* 6:41–51, 1960

39. Korst DR, Johnson D, Frenkel EP, et al: Preliminary evaluation of the effect of cyclophosphamide on the course of human neoplasms. *Cancer Chemother Rep* 7:1–12, 1960

40. Papac R, Petrakis NL, Amini F, et al: Comparative clinical evaluation of two alkylating agents (mannitol mustard and cyclophosphamide). *JAMA* 172:1387–1391, 1960

41. Hoogstraten B, Schroeder LR, Freireich EJ, et al: Cyclophosphamide

(Cytoxan) in acute leukemia: Preliminary report. *Cancer Chemother Rep* 8:116–119, 1960

42. *Physicians' Desk Reference*, ed. 44. Oradell, NJ, Medical Economics Co., 1990.
43. Brock N: Pharmakologische Untersuchungen mit neuen N-chloroäthyl-phosphorsäureester-diamiden. In *Proceedings of the Fifth International Congress of Chemotherapy*, vol. 2, Spitzy KH, Haschek H (eds.). Vienna, Verlag der Wiener Medizinischen Akademie, pp. 155–161, 1967
44. Cohen MH, Mittelman A: Initial clinical trial of isofosfamide (abstract). *Proc Am Assoc Cancer Res* 14:64, 1973
45. Brock N: Pharmacological studies with ifosfamide: A new oxazaphosphorine compound (Proceedings of the Seventh International Congress of Chemotherapy, Prague, 1971). In *Advances in Antimicrobial and Antineoplastic Chemotherapy*, vol. 2, Semonský M, Hejzler M, Masák S (eds.). Baltimore, University Park Press, pp. 749–756, 1972
46. Scheef W: Problems, experience, and results of clinical investigations with ifosfamide (Proceedings of the Seventh International Congress of Chemotherapy, Prague, 1971). In *Advances in Antimicrobial and Antineoplastic Chemotherapy*, vol. 2, Semonský M, Hejzler M, Masák S (eds.). Baltimore, University Park Press, pp. 797–800, 1972
47. van Dyk JJ, Falkson HC, van der Merwe AM, et al: Unexpected toxicity in patients treated with iphosphamide. *Cancer Res* 32:921–924, 1972
48. Rodriguez V, Bodey GP, Freireich EJ, et al: Reduction of ifosfamide toxicity using dose fractionation. *Cancer Res* 36:2945–2948, 1976
49. Rodriguez V, McCredie KB, Keating MJ, et al: Isophosphamide therapy for hematologic malignancies in patients refractory to prior treatment. *Cancer Treat Rep* 62:493–497, 1978
50. Brock N, Pohl J, Stekar J: Studies on the urotoxicity of oxazaphosphorine cytostatics and its prevention: 1. Experimental studies on the urotoxicity of alkylating compounds. *Eur J Cancer Clin Oncol* 17:596–607, 1981
51. Brock N, Pohl J, Stekar J: Studies on the urotoxicity of oxazaphosphorine cytostatics and its prevention: III. Profile of action of sodium 2-mercaptoethane sulfonate (mesna). *Eur J Cancer Clin Oncol* 18:1377–1387, 1982
52. Scheef W, Klein HD, Brock N, et al: Controlled clinical studies with an antidote against the urotoxicity of oxazaphosphorines: Preliminary results. *Cancer Treat Rep* 63:501–505, 1979
53. Case DC Jr, Anderson J, Ervin TJ, et al: Phase II trial of ifosfamide and mesna in previously treated patients with non-Hodgkin's lymphoma: Cancer and Leukemia Group B study. *Med Pediatr Oncol* 16:182–186, 1988
54. Norberg B, Holm J, Winqvist E, et al: Treatment of advanced bone marrow neoplasms with ifosfamide combinations. *Scand J Haematol* 32:95–100, 1984
55. Ryan DH, Kopecky KJ, Head D, et al: Phase II evaluation of teniposide

and ifosfamide in refractory adult acute lymphocytic leukemia: A Southwest Oncology Group study. *Cancer Treat Rep* 71:713–716, 1987

56. Huggins C, Hodges CV: Studies on prostate cancer: I. The effect of castration, of estrogen and of androgen injection on serum phosphatases in metastatic carcinoma of the prostate. *Cancer Res* 1:293–297, 1941

57. Dougherty TF, White A. Effect of pituitary adrenotropic hormone on lymphoid tissue. *Proc Soc Exp Biol Med* 53:132–133, 1943

58. Ingle DJ: Atrophy of the thymus in normal and hypophysectomized rats following administration of cortin. *Proc Soc Exp Biol Med* 38:443–444, 1938

59. Rosenthal MC, Saunders RH, Schwartz LI, et al: The use of adrenocorticotropic hormone and cortisone in the treatment of leukemia and leukosarcoma. *Blood* 6:804–823, 1951

60. Pearson OH, Eliel LP, Rawson RW, et al: ACTH- and cortisone-induced regression of lymphoid tumors in man. *Cancer* 2:943–945, 1949

61. Farber S, Shwachman H, Toch R, et al: The effect of ACTH in acute leukemia in childhood. In *Proceedings of the First Clinical ACTH Conference*, Mote JR (ed.). Philadelphia, Blakiston, pp. 328–330, 1950

62. Haddow A, Sexton WA: Influence of carbamic esters (urethanes) on experimental animal tumours. *Nature* 157:500–503, 1946

63. Paterson E, ApThomas I, Haddow A, et al: Leukemia treated with urethane compared with deep x-ray therapy. *Lancet* 1:677–683, 1946

64. Leuchtenberger C, Lewisohn R, Laszlo D, et al: "Folic acid," a tumor growth inhibitor. *Proc Soc Exp Biol Med* 55:204–205, 1944

65. Leuchtenberger R, Leuchtenberger C, Laszlo D, et al: The influence of "folic acid" on spontaneous breast cancer in mice. *Science* 101:46, 1945

66. Farber S: Action of pteroylglutamine conjugates on man. *Science* 106:619–621, 1947

67. Heinle RW, Welch AD: Experiments with pteroylglutamine acid and pteroylglutamine acid deficiency in human leukemia (abstract). *J Clin Invest* 27:539, 1948

68. Farber S: Some observations on the effect of folic acid antagonists on acute leukemia and other forms of incurable cancer. *Blood* 4:160–167, 1949

69. Farber S, Diamond LK, Mercer RD, et al: Temporary remissions in acute leukemia in children prolonged by folic acid antagonist, 4-aminopteroylglutamic acid (aminopterin). *N Engl J Med* 238:787–793, 1948

70. Li MC, Hertz R, Spencer DB: Effect of methotrexate upon choriocarcinoma and chorioadenoma. *Proc Soc Exp Biol Med* 93:361–366, 1956

71. Law LW, Dunn TB, Boyle PJ, et al: Observations on the effect of a folic acid antagonist on transplantable lymphoid leukemias in mice. *JNCI* 10:179–192, 1949

72. Rieselbach RE, Morse EE, Rall DP, et al: Intrathecal aminopterin therapy of meningeal leukemia. *Arch Intern Med* 111:620–630, 1963

73. Rall DP, Rieselbach RE, Oliverio VT, et al: Pharmacology of folic acid antagonists as related to brain and cerebrospinal fluid. *Cancer Chemother Rep* 16:187–190, 1962

74. Hitchings GH, Elion GB: The chemistry and biochemistry of purine analogs. *Ann NY Acad Sci* 60:195–199, 1954
75. Law LW: Resistance in leukemic cells to an adenine antagonist, 6-MP. *Proc Soc Exp Biol Med* 84:409–412, 1953
76. Clarke DA, Philips FS, Sternberg SS, et al: 6-Mercaptopurine: Effects in mouse sarcoma 180 and in normal animals. *Cancer Res* 13:593–604, 1953
77. Burchenal JH, Murphy ML, Ellison RR, et al: Clinical evaluation of a new antimetabolite, 6-mercaptopurine, in the treatment of leukemia and allied diseases. *Blood* 8:965–999, 1953
78. Bergmann W, Feeney R: Contributions to the study of marine products: XXXII. The nucleosides of sponges. *J Organic Chem* 16:981–987, 1951
79. Bergmann W, Burke DC: Contributions to the study of marine products: XXXIX. The nucleosides of sponges. III: Spongothymidine and spongouridine. *J Organic Chem* 20:1501–1507, 1955
80. Pizer LI, Cohen SS: Metabolism of pyrimidine arabinonucleosides and cyclonucleosides in *Escherichia coli. J Biol Chem* 235:2387–2392, 1960
81. Chabner BA: Cytosine arabinoside. In *Pharmacologic Principles of Cancer Treatment.* Philadelphia, W.B. Saunders, pp. 387–401, 1982
82. Walwick ER, Roberts WK, Dekker CA: Cyclisation during the phosphorylation of uridine and cytidine by polyphosphoric acid: A new route to the $O^2,2'$-cyclonucleosides. In *Proceedings. Chemical Society (London) 84, March 1959. Chem Abstr* 53:21982d, November 1959
83. Chu MY, Fischer GA: A proposed mechanism of action of 1-β-D-arabinofuranosyl-cytosine as an inhibitor of the growth of leukemic cells. *Biochem Pharmacol* 11:423–430, 1962
84. Chu MY, Fischer GA: Comparative studies of leukemic cells sensitive and resistant to cytosine arabinoside. *Biochem Pharmacol* 14:333–341, 1965
85. Cohen SS: Introduction to the biochemistry of D-arabinosyl nucleosides. *Prog Nucleic Acid Res Mol Biol* 5:1–88, 1966
86. Evans JS, Musser EA, Mengel GD, et al: Antitumor activity of l-β-D-arabinofuranosylcytosine hydrochloride. *Proc Soc Exp Biol Med* 106:350–353, 1961
87. Talley RW, Vaitkevicius VK: Megaloblastosis produced by a cytosine antagonist 1-β-D-arabinofuranosylcytosine. *Blood* 21:352–362, 1963
88. Schabel FM Jr, Skipper HE, Trader MW, et al: Experimental evaluation of potential anticancer agents: XIX. Sensitivity of nondividing leukemic cell populations to certain classes of drugs in vivo. *Cancer Chemother Rep* 48:17–30, 1965
89. Skipper HE, Schabel FM Jr, Wilcox WS: Experimental evaluation of potential anticancer agents: XXI. Scheduling of arabinosylcytosine to take advantage of its S-phase specificity against leukemic cells. *Cancer Chemother Rep* 51:125–141, 1967
90. Freireich EJ, Bodey GP, Harris JE, et al: Therapy for acute granulocytic leukemia. *Cancer Res* 27:2573–2577, 1967
91. Ellison RR, Holland JF, Silver RT, et al. Cytosine arabinoside: A new

drug for induction of remissions in acute leukemia. In *Abstracts of the Ninth International Cancer Congress (Tokyo)*, p. 645, 1966

92. Wilmanns W, Mainzer K, Müller D, et al: The treatment of acute leukaemia with cytosine arabinoside: Biochemical and clinical findings. *German Med Monthly* 14:317–324, 1969

93. Ellison RR, Holland JF, Weil M, et al: Arabinosyl cytosine: Useful agent in the treatment of acute leukemia in adults. *Blood* 32:507–521, 1968

94. Frei E III, Bickers JN, Hewlett JS, et al: Dose schedule and antitumor studies of arabinosyl cytosine. *Cancer Res* 29:1325–1332, 1969

95. Southwest Oncology Group: Cytarabine for acute leukemia in adults. *Arch Intern Med* 133:251–259, 1974

96. Freireich EJ: Arabinosyl cytosine: A 20-year update. *J Clin Oncol* 5:523–524, 1987

97. Estey E, Keating M, Plunkett W, et al: High-dose continuous infusion cytosine arabinoside (ara-C) without anthracycline produces high CR rates in adults under age 50 with previously untreated AML (abstract). *Blood* 58:2220, 1986

98. Capizzi RL, Poole M, Cooper MR, et al: Treatment of poor risk acute leukemia with sequential high-dose Ara-C and asparaginase. *Blood* 63:694–700, 1984

99. Rudnick SA, Cadman EC, Capizzi RL, et al: High dose cytosine arabinoside (HDARAC) in refractory acute leukemia. *Cancer* 44:1189–1193, 1979

100. Karanes C, Wolff SN, Herzig GP, et al: High dose cytosine arabinoside (Ara-C) in the treatment of patients (Pts) with refractory acute non-lymphocytic leukemia (ANLL) (abstract). *Blood* 54(Suppl):191a, 1979

101. Herzig RH, Wolff SN, Lazarus HM, et al: High-dose cytosine arabinoside for refractory leukemia. *Blood* 62:361–369, 1983

102. Preisler HD, Epstein J, Barcos M, et al: Prediction of response of acute nonlymphocytic leukaemia to therapy with 'high dose' cytosine arabinoside. *Br J Haematol* 58:19–32, 1984

103. Keating MJ, Estey E, Plunkett W, et al: Evolution of clinical studies with high-dose cytosine arabinoside at the M. D. Anderson Hospital. *Semin Oncol* 12(Suppl 3):98–104, 1985

104. *Dorland's Illustrated Medical Dictionary*, ed. 26. Philadelphia, W.B. Saunders, 1985

105. Lang S: Über Desamidierung im Tierkorper. *Beitr Chem Physiol Pathol* 5:321–345, 1904

106. Clementi A: La désamidation enzymatique de L-asparagine chez les differentes espèces animales et la signification physiologique de sa présence dans l'organisme. *Arch Int Physiol* 19:369–398, 1922

107. Kidd JG: Regression of transplanted lymphomas induced in vivo by means of normal guinea pig serum: I. Course of transplanted cancers of various kinds in mice and rats given guinea pig serum, horse serum or rabbit serum. *J Exp Med* 98:565–582, 1953

108. Broome JD: Evidence that the L-asparaginase activity of guinea pig serum is responsible for its antilymphoma effects. *Nature* 191:1114–1115, 1961

109. Old LJ, Boyse EA, Campbell HA, et al: Leukaemia-inhibiting properties and L-asparaginase activity of sera from certain South American rodents. *Nature* 198:801, 1963

110. Old LJ, Boyse EA, Campbell HA, et al: Treatment of lymphosarcoma in the dog with L-asparaginase. *Cancer* 20:1066–1070, 1967

111. Dolowy WC, Henson D, Cornet J, et al: Toxic and anti-neoplastic effects of L-asparaginase: Study of mice with lymphoma and normal monkeys and report on a child with leukemia. *Cancer* 19:1813–1819, 1966

112. Hill JM, Roberts J, Loeb E, et al: L-Asparaginase therapy for leukemia and other malignant neoplasms: Remission in human leukemia. *JAMA* 202:882–888, 1967

113. Oettgen HF, Old LJ, Boyse EA, et al: Inhibition of leukemias in man by L-asparaginase. *Cancer Res* 27:2619–2631, 1967

114. Johnson IS, Wright HF, Svoboda GH, et al: Antitumor principles derived from *Vinca rosea* Linn: I. Vincaleukoblastine and leurosine. *Cancer Res* 20:1016–1022, 1960

115. Peckolt T: Heil- und Nutzpflanzen braziliens. *Beitr Dtsch Pharmazeutischen Ges* 20:36–58, 1910

116. Perrot E: *Matières premières uselles du regne vegetal*, ed. 1. Paris, Masson et cie, p. 1783, 1943–44

117. Noble RL, Beer CT, Cutts JH: Role of chance observations in chemotherapy: *Vinca rosea*. *Ann NY Acad Sci* 76:882–894, 1958

118. Garcia F: A botany symposium on medicinal plants. In *Proceedings of the Eighth Pacific Science Congress of the Pacific Science Association*, vol. 4. Manila, National Research Council of the Philippines, p. 182, 1954

119. Johnson IS, Wright HF, Svoboda GH: Experimental basis for clinical evaluation of anti-tumor principles derived from *Vinca rosea* Linn (abstract). *J Lab Clin Med* 54:830, 1959

120. Cutts JH, Beer CT, Noble RL: Biologic properties of vinca-leukoblastine, an alkaloid in *Vinca rosea* Linn, with reference to its antitumor actions. *Cancer Res* 20:1023–1031, 1960

121. Hodes ME, Rohn RJ, Bond W: Effects of a plant alkaloid, vincaleukoblastine, in human beings (abstract). *J Lab Clin Med* 54:826, 1959

122. Karon MR, Freireich EJ, Frei E III: A preliminary report on vincristine sulfate: A new active agent for the treatment of acute leukemia. *Pediatrics* 30:791–796, 1962

123. Carbone PP, Bono V, Frei E III, et al: Clinical studies with vincristine. *Blood* 21:640–647, 1963

124. Selawry OS, Frei E III: Prolongation of remission in acute lymphocytic leukemia by alteration in dose schedule and route of administration of methotrexate (abstract). *Clin Res* 12:231, 1964

125. Burgess MA, Garson OM, DeGrunchy GC: Daunorubicin in the treatment of adult acute leukaemia. *Med J Aust* 1:629–635, 1970

126. Grein A, Spalla C, DiMarco A: Descrizione e classificazione di un attimomycite (*Streptomyces peucetius sp. Nova*) produttoce di una sos-

taviza ad attivita antitumorale—La daunomicina. *G Microbiol* 11:109, 1963

127. DuBost M, Ganter P, Maral R, et al: Un nouvel antibiotique à propriétès antitumorales. *C R Acad Sci [III]* 257:1813–1820, 1963

128. DiMarco A, Gaetani M, Orezzi P, et al: Antitumor activity of a new antibiotic: Daunomycin. In *Proceedings of the Third International Congress of Chemotherapy*, vol. 2. Stuttgart, 1963, New York, Hafner, pp. 1023–1031, 1964

129. DiMarco A, Gaetani M, Orezzi P, et al: "Daunomycin," a new antibiotic of the rhodomycin group. *Nature* 201:706–707, 1964

130. DuBost M, Ganter P, Maral R, et al: Rubidomycin: A new antibiotic with cytostatic properties. *Cancer Chemother Rep* 41:35–36, 1964

131. Jacquillat C, Boiron M, Weil M, et al: Rubidomycin: A new agent active in the treatment of acute lymphoblastic leukemia. *Lancet* 2:27–28, 1966

132. Howard JP, Tan C: Combined daunomycin-prednisone inductions in acute leukemia (abstract). *Proc Am Assoc Cancer Res* 8:32, 1967

133. Holton CP, Lonsdale D, Nora AH, et al: Clinical study of daunomycin in children with acute leukemia. *Cancer* 22:1014–1018, 1968

134. Holton CP, Vietti TJ, Nora AH, et al: Clinical study of daunomycin and prednisone for induction of remission in children with advanced leukemia. *N Engl J Med* 280:171–174, 1969

135. Dano K: Development of resistance to Adriamycin in Ehrlich ascites tumor in vivo. *Cancer Chemother Rep* 56:321–326, 1972

136. Bonadonna G, Monfardini S, De Lena M, et al: Phase I and preliminary phase II evaluation of Adriamycin. *Cancer Res* 30:2572–2582, 1970

137. DiMarco A, Gaetani M, Scarpinato B: Adriamycin: A new antibiotic with antitumor activity. *Cancer Chemother Rep* 53:33–37, 1969

138. Carter SK: Adriamycin: A review. *JNCI* 55:1265–1274, 1975

139. McCredie KB, Bodey GP, Gutterman JU, et al: Sequential Adriamycin-Ara-C (A-OAP) for remission induction (RI) of adult acute leukemia (AAL) (abstract). *Proc Am Assoc Cancer Res* 15:62, 1974

140. Mellanby E: Suppression of oxygen uptake of cancerous growths. In *British Empire Cancer Campaign for Research, 10th Annual Report.* Hampshire, England, Macmillan, pp. 102–104, 1933

141. Von Hoff DD, Howser D, Gormley P, et al: Phase I study of methane-sulfonamide, N-[4-(9-acridinylamino)-3-methoxyphenyl]-(m-AMSA) using a single-dose schedule. *Cancer Treat Rep* 62:1421–1426, 1978

142. Cain BF, Atwell GJ: The experimental antitumour properties of three congeners of the acridylmethanesulphonanilide (AMSA) series. *Eur J Cancer* 10:539–549, 1974

143. Gormley PE, Sethi VS, Cysyk RL: Interaction of 4'-(9-acridinylamino) methanesulfon-m-anisidide with DNA and inhibition of oncornavirus reverse transcriptase and cellular nucleic acid polymerases. *Cancer Res* 38:1300–1306, 1978

144. Tewey KM, Chen GL, Nelson EM, et al: Intercalative antitumor drugs interfere with the breakage-reunion reaction of mammalian DNA topoisomerase II. *J Biol Chem* 259:9182–9187, 1984

145. Nelson EM, Tewey KM, Liu LF, et al: Mechanism of antitumor drug action: Poisoning of mammalian DNA topoisomerase II on DNA by 4'-(9-acridinylamino)-methanesulfon-*m*-anisidide. *Proc Natl Acad Sci USA* 81:1361–1365, 1984

146. Legha SS, Gutterman JU, Hall SW, et al: Phase I clinical investigation of 4'-(9-acridinylamino) methanesulfon-*m*-aniside (NSC 249992), a new acridine derivative. *Cancer Res* 38:3712–3716, 1978

147. Legha SS, Keating MJ, Zander AR, et al: 4'(9-acridinylamino) methanesulfon-*m*-aniside (AMSA): A new drug effective in the treatment of adult acute leukemia. *Ann Intern Med* 93:17–21, 1980

148. Legha SS, Keating MJ, McCredie KB, et al: Evaluation of AMSA in previously treated patients with acute leukemia: Results of therapy in 109 adults. *Blood* 60:484–490, 1982

149. Peters WG, Willemze R, Colly LP: Results of induction and consolidation treatment with intermediate and high-dose cytosine arabinoside and m-AMSA of patients with poor-risk acute myelogenous leukaemia. *Eur J Haematol* 40:198–204, 1988

150. Dhaliwal HS, Shannon MS, Barnett MJ, et al: Treatment of acute leukaemia with m-AMSA in combination with cytosine arabinoside. *Cancer Chemother Pharmacol* 18:59–62, 1986

151. Arlin ZA, Gee TS, Kempin SJ, et al: Treatment of adult non-lymphoblastic leukemia (ANLL) with AMSA in combination with cytosine arabinoside (Ara-C) and 6-thioguanine (AAT) (abstract). *Proc Am Assoc Cancer Res* 22:172, 1981

152. McCredie KB, Keating MJ, Estey EH, et al: Use of a 4'(9-acridinylamino) methanesulfon-*m*-anisidide (AMSA), cytosine-arabinoside (Ara-C), vincristine, prednisone combination (AMSA-OAP) in poor-risk patients in acute leukemia (abstract). *Proc Am Soc Clin Oncol* 22:479, 1981

153. Estey EH, Keating MJ, Smith TL, et al: Prediction of complete remission in patients with refractory acute leukemia treated with AMSA. *J Clin Oncol* 2:102–106, 1984

154. Freireich EJ: New strategies in the management of acute leukemia. *Acta Haematol* 78(Suppl 1):116–119, 1987

155. Kaplan IW: Condylomata acuminata. *New Orleans Med Surg J* 94:388–390, 1942

156. Kelly MG, Hartwell JL: The biological effects and the chemical composition of podophyllin: A review. *JNCI* 14:967–1010, 1954

157. Stähelin H: 4'-Demethyl-epipodophyllotoxin thenylidene glucoside (VM 26), a podophyllum compound with a new mechanism of action. *Eur J Cancer* 6:303–311, 1970

158. Cornman I, Cornman ME: The action of podophyllin and its fractions on marine eggs. *Ann NY Acad Sci* 51:1443–1487, 1951

159. Greenspan EM, Leiter J, Shear MJ: Effect of alpha-peltatin, beta-peltatin, and podophyllotoxin on lymphoma and other transplanted tumors. *JNCI* 10:1295–1317, 1950

160. Vaitkevicius VK, Reed ML: Clinical studies with podophyllum compounds SPI-77 (NSC-72274) and SPG-827 (NSC-42076). *Cancer Chemother Rep* 50:565–571, 1966

161. Dombernowsky P, Nissen NI: Schedule dependency of the antileukemic activity of the podophyllotoxin-derivative VP–16–213 (NSC 141540) in L1210 leukemia. *Acta Pathol Microbiol Scand* 81A:715–724, 1973

162. EORTC Clinical Screening Group: Epipodophyllotoxin VP 16 213 in treatment of acute leukaemias, haematosarcomas, and solid tumours. *Br Med J* 3:199–202, 1973

163. Rivera G, Avery T, Pratt C: 4'-Demethylepipodophyllotoxin 9-(4,6-O-2-thenylidene-β-D-glucopyranoside) (NSC–122819; VM–26) and 4'demethyl-epipodophyllotoxin 9-(4,6-O-ethylidene-β-D-glucopyranoside) (NSC–141540; VP–16–213) in childhood cancer: Preliminary observations. *Cancer Chemother Rep* 59:743–749, 1975

164. Radice PA, Bunn PA Jr, Ihde DC: Therapeutic trials with VP–16–213 and VM–26: Active agents in small cell lung cancer, non-Hodgkin's lymphomas, and other malignancies. *Cancer Treat Rep* 63:1231–1239, 1979

165. Chard RL Jr, Krivit W, Bleyer WA, et al: Phase II study of VP–16–213 in childhood malignant disease: A Children's Cancer Study Group report. *Cancer Treat Rep* 63:1755–1759, 1979

166. Rivera G, Murphy SB, Wood A, et al: Combination chemotherapy with prednisone, vincristine and the epipodophyllotoxin VM–26 for refractory childhood lymphocytic leukemia (ALL) (abstract). *Blood* 54:205a, 1979

167. Rivera G, Dahl GV, Bowman WP, et al: VM–26 and cytosine arabinoside combination chemotherapy for initial induction failures in childhood lymphocytic leukemia. *Cancer* 46:1727–1730, 1980

168. Blume KG, Forman SJ: High dose busulfan/etoposide as a preparatory regimen for second bone marrow transplants in hematologic malignancies. *Blut* 55:49–53, 1987

169. Kushner BH, Kwon J-H, Gulati SC, et al: Preclinical assessment of purging with VP–16–213: Key role for long-term marrow cultures. *Blood* 69:65–71, 1987

170. Pui C-H, Behm FG, Raimondi SC, et al: Secondary acute myeloid leukemia in children treated for acute lymphoid leukemia. *N Engl J Med* 321:136–142, 1989

171. Civin CI: Reducing the cost of the cure of childhood leukemia. *N Engl J Med* 321:185–187, 1989

172. Murdock KC, Child RG, Fabio PF, et al: Antitumor agents: I. 1,4-bis[(aminoalkyl) amino]–9,10-anthracenediones. *J Med Chem* 22:1024–1030, 1979

173. Zee-Cheng RK-Y, Cheng CC: Antineoplastic agents: Structure-activity relationship study of bis(substituted aminoalkylamino) anthraquinones. *J Med Chem* 21:291–294, 1978

174. Smith IE: Mitoxantrone (Novantrone): A review of experimental and early clinical studies. *Cancer Treat Rev* 10:103–115, 1983

175. Adamson RH: Daunomycin (NSC–82151) and Adriamycin (NSC–123127): A hypothesis concerning antitumor activity and cardiotoxicity. *Cancer Chemother Rep* 58:293–294, 1974

176. Bergsagel DE: Introduction to the symposium. New Perspectives in

Chemotherapy: Focus on Novantrone, Toronto, Canada. February 23, 1984, Semin Oncol 11(3 Suppl 1):1–2, 1984

177. Vietti T, Nix W, Kim T, et al: Dianhydroanthracenedione (DA) in children (C) with advanced malignant disease: A POG and American Cyanamid phase I study (abstract). Proc Am Assoc Cancer Res 22:237, 1981

178. Estey EH, Keating MJ, McCredie KB, et al: Phase II trial of mitoxantrone in refractory acute leukemia. Cancer Treat Rep 67:389–390, 1983

179. Arlin ZA, Dukart G, Schoch I, et al: Phase I–II trial of mitoxantrone in acute leukemia: An interim report. Invest New Drugs 3:213–217, 1985

180. Starling KA, Mulne AF, Vats TS, et al: Mitoxantrone in refractory acute leukemia in children: A phase I study. Invest New Drugs 3:191–195, 1985

181. Shenkenberg TD, Von Hoff DD: Mitoxantrone: A new anticancer drug with significant clinical activity. Ann Intern Med 105:67–81, 1986

182. Bollag W, Grunberg E: Tumor inhibitory effects of a new class of cytotoxic agents: Methylhydrazine derivatives. Experientia 19:130–131, 1963

183. Oliverio VT: Derivatives of triazenes and hydrazines. In Cancer Medicine, Holland JF, Frei E III (eds.). Philadelphia, Lea & Febiger, pp. 850–860, 1982

184. Zeller P, Gutmann H, Hegedus B, et al: Methylhydrazine derivatives, a new class of cytotoxic agents. Experientia 19:129, 1963

185. Reed JD: Procarbazine. In Handbook of Experimental Pharmacology, Antineoplastic and Immunosuppressive Agents, Part II, Sartorelli AC, Johns DG (eds.). Berlin, Springer-Verlag, pp. 747–765, 1975

186. Berneis K, Kofler M, Bollag W, et al: The degradation of deoxyribonucleic acid by new tumor inhibiting compounds: The intermediate formation of hydrogen peroxide. Experientia 19:132–133, 1963

187. Frei E III: Summary and perspectives. In Hodgkin's Disease and Non-Hodgkin's Lymphoma: University of Texas M. D. Anderson Clinical Conference on Cancer, vol. 27, Ford RJ Jr, Fuller LM, Hagemeister FB (eds.). New York, Raven Press, pp. 427–434, 1983

188. Thiele J, Dralle E: Zur Kenntnis des Amidoguanidins: I. Condensations-Produkte des Amidoguanidins mit Aldehyden und Ketonen der Fettreihe. Ann Chem 302:275–299, 1898

189. Warrell RP Jr, Burchenal JH: Methylglyoxal-bis(guanylhydrazone) (methyl-GAG): Current status and future prospects. J Clin Oncol 1:52–65, 1983

190. Freedlander BL, French FA: Carcinostatic action of polycarbonyl compounds and their derivatives: I. 3-Ethoxy–2-ketobutyraldehyde and related compounds. Cancer Res 18:172–175, 1958

191. Freedlander BL, French FA: Carcinostatic action of polycarbonyl compounds and their derivatives: II. Glyoxal bis(guanylhydrazone) and derivatives. Cancer Res 18:360–363, 1958

192. Freedlander BL, French FA: Hydroxymethylglyoxal bis(guanylhydrazone). Cancer Res 18:1286–1289, 1958

193. Freedlander BL, French FA: Glyoxal bis(thiosemicarbazone) and derivatives. Cancer Res 18:1290–1300, 1958

194. Corti A, Dave C, Williams-Ashman HG: Specific inhibition of the enzymic decarboxylation of *S*-adenosylmethionine by methylglyoxal bis(guanylhydrazone) and related substances. *Biochem J* 139:351–357, 1974

195. Warrell RP Jr, Lee BJ, Kempin SJ, et al: Effectiveness of methyl-GAG (methylglyoxal-bis(guanylhydrazone)) in patients with advanced malignant lymphoma. *Blood* 57:1011–1014, 1981

196. Pine M, DePaolo J: The antimitochrondrial action of 2-chloro–4',4"-bis(2-imidazolin–2-yl) terephtalanilide and methylglyoxal-bis (guanylhydrazone). *Cancer Res* 26:18–25, 1966

197. Sartorelli AC, Iannotti AT, Booth BA, et al: Complex formation with DNA and inhibition of nucleic acid synthesis by methylglyoxal bis(guanylhydrazone). *Biochem Biophys Acta* 103:174–176, 1965

198. Regelson W, Holland JF: Initial clinical study of parenteral methylglyoxal bis(guanylhydrazone) diacetate. *Cancer Chemother Rep* 11:81–86, 1961

199. Freireich EJ, Frei E III, Karon M: Methylglyoxal-bis(guanylhydrazone): A new agent active against acute myelocytic leukemia. *Cancer Chemother Rep* 16:183–186, 1962

200. Carbone PP, Freireich EJ, Frei E III, et al: The effectiveness of methylglyoxal-bis-guanylhydrazone (CH$_3$-G) in human malignant disease. *Acta Unio Internationalis Contra Cancrum* 20:340–343, 1964

201. Mihich E: Current studies with methylglyoxal-bis(guanylhydrazone). *Cancer Res* 23:1375–1389, 1963

202. Knight WA III, Livingston RB, Fabian C, et al: Phase I-II trial of methyl-GAG: A Southwest Oncology Group pilot study. *Cancer Treat Rep* 63:1933–1937, 1979

203. Pinkel D: Curing children of leukemia. *Accomplishments Cancer Res* 2:57–72, 1986

5. Adjuvant, Maintenance, and Combination Chemotherapy

1. Furth J, Kahn MC: The transmission of leukemia of mice with a single cell. *Am J Cancer* 31:276–282, 1937

2. Perloff M, Holland JF, Frei E III: Adjuvant chemotherapy. In *Cancer Medicine*, Holland JF, Frei E III (eds.). Philadelphia, Lea & Febiger, pp. 515–527, 1982

3. Osgood EE, Seaman AJ: Treatment of chronic leukemia. *JAMA* 150:1372–1379, 1952

4. Smith CH, Bell WR: Aminopterin in treatment of leukemia in children. *Am J Dis Child* 79:1031–1048, 1950

5. Farber S: *Proc Div Lab Res* 1:1–5 (The Children's Medical Center, Boston), 1948

6. Farber S, Toch R, Sears EM, et al: Advances in chemotherapy of cancer in man. *Adv Cancer Res* 4:1–71, 1956

7. Zubrod CG: Historic milestones in curative chemotherapy. *Semin Oncol* 6:490–505, 1979

8. Farber S, D'Angio G, Evans A, et al: Clinical studies of actinomycin D

with special reference to Wilms' tumor in children. *Ann NY Acad Sci* 89:421–425, 1960

9. D'Angio GJ, Farber S, Maddock CL: Potentiation of x-ray effects by actinomycin D. *Radiology* 73:175–177, 1959

10. Cruz EP, McDonald GO, Cole WH: Prophylactic treatment of cancer: The use of chemotherapeutic agents to prevent tumor metastases. *Surgery* 40:291–296, 1956

11. Shimkin MB, Moore GE: Adjuvant use of chemotherapy in the surgical treatment of cancer. *JAMA* 167:1710–1714, 1958

12. Freireich EJ, Gehan EA, Frei E III: The effect of 6-mercaptopurine on the duration of steroid-induced remissions in acute leukemia: A model for evaluation of other potentially useful therapy. *Blood* 21:699–716, 1963

13. Freireich EJ, Frei E III: Recent advances in acute leukemia. *Prog Hematol* 4:187–202, 1964

14. Skipper HE, Schabel FM, Jay R, et al: Experimental evaluation of potential antitumor agents: On the criteria and kinetics associated with curability of experimental leukemia. *Cancer Chemother Rep* 35:1–111, 1964

15. Frei E III: Acute leukemia in children. *Cancer* 53:2013–2025, 1984

16. Frei E III, Freireich EJ: Progress and perspectives in the chemotherapy of acute leukemia. *Adv Chemother* 2:269–289, 1965

17. Skipper HE: Carbamates in the chemotherapy of leukemia. V. Observation of a possible antileukemic synergism between urethane and methylbis(β-chloroethyl)amine. *Cancer* 2:475–479, 1949

18. Law LW: Effects of combinations of antileukemic agents on an acute lymphocytic leukemia of mice. *Cancer Res* 12:871–878, 1952

19. Skipper HE, Thomson JR, Bell M: Attempts at dual blocking of biochemical events in cancer chemotherapy. *Cancer Res* 14:503–507, 1954

20. Potter VR: Sequential blocking of metabolic pathways in vivo. *Proc Soc Exp Biol Med* 76:41–46, 1951

21. Elion GB, Singer S, Hitchings GH: Antagonists of nucleic acid derivatives: Synergism in combinations of biochemically related antimetabolites. *J Biol Chem* 208:477–488, 1954

22. Clarke DA, Phillips FS, Buckley SM, et al: Presented at the 125th Meeting of American Chemical Society, Kansas City, March 1954

23. Frei E III, Holland JF, Schneiderman MA, et al: A comparative study of two regimens of combination chemotherapy in acute leukemia. *Blood* 13:1126–1148, 1958

24. Hill AB: The clinical trial. *N Engl J Med* 247:113–119, 1952

25. Frei E III, Freireich EJ, Gehan E, et al: Studies of sequential and combination antimetabolite therapy in acute leukemia: 6-mercaptopurine and methotrexate. *Blood* 18:431–454, 1961

26. Blum RH, Frei E III, Holland JF: Principles of dose, schedule, and combination chemotherapy. In *Cancer Medicine*, Holland JF, Frei E III (eds.). Philadelphia, Lea & Febiger, pp. 730–752, 1982

27. Frei E III, Karon M, Levin RH, et al: The effectiveness of combinations of antileukemic agents in inducing and maintaining remission in children with acute leukemia. *Blood* 26:642–656, 1965

28. Acute Leukemia Group B: New treatment schedule with improved survival in childhood leukemia. *JAMA* 194:75–81, 1965
29. Freireich EJ, Gehan EA, Sulman D, et al: The effect of chemotherapy in acute leukemia in the human. *J Chronic Dis* 14:593–608, 1961
30. Zubrod CG: The Fifth Myron Karon Memorial Lecture: The cure of cancer by chemotherapy—reflections on how it happened *Med Pediatr Oncol* 8:107–114, 1980
31. Freireich EJ, Henderson ES, Karon MR, et al: The treatment of acute leukemia considered with respect to cell population kinetics. In *The Proliferation and Spread of Neoplastic Cells, 21st Annual Symposium on Fundamental Cancer Research (The University of Texas M. D. Anderson Hospital & Tumor Institute at Houston).* Baltimore, Williams & Wilkins, pp. 441–452, 1968
32. Freireich EJ, Karon M, Frei E III: Quadruple combination therapy (VAMP) for acute lymphocytic leukemia of childhood (abstract). *Proc Am Assoc Cancer Res* 5:20, 1964
33. Freireich EJ, Karon M, Flatow F, et al: Effect of intensive cyclic chemotherapy (BIKE) on remission duration in acute lymphocytic leukemia (abstract). *Proc Am Assoc Cancer Res* 6:20, 1965
34. Henderson ES: Combination chemotherapy of acute lymphocytic leukemia of childhood. *Cancer Res* 27:2570–2572, 1967
35. Pinkel D: Five-year follow-up of "total therapy" of childhood lymphocytic leukemia. *JAMA* 216:648–652, 1971
36. Pinkel D: Curing children of leukemia. *Accomplishments Cancer Res* 2:57–72, 1986
37. DeVita VT, Moxley JH III, Brace KC, et al: Intensive combination chemotherapy and x-irradiation in the treatment of Hodgkin's disease (abstract). *Proc Am Assoc Cancer Res* 6:15, 1965
38. Zubrod CG: Origins and development of chemotherapy research at the National Cancer Institute. *Cancer Treat Rep* 68:9–19, 1984
39. DeVita VT, Serpick AA, Carbone PP: Combination chemotherapy in the treatment of advanced Hodgkin's disease. *Ann Intern Med* 73:881–895, 1970
40. DeVita V, Canellos G, Hubbard S, et al: Chemotherapy of Hodgkin's disease (HD) with MOPP: A 10-year progress report (abstract). *Proc Am Assoc Cancer Res Am Soc Clin Oncol* 17:269, 1976
41. Freireich EJ, Keating M, Cabanillas F, et al: The hematologic malignancies: Leukemia, lymphoma, and myeloma. *Cancer* 54:2741–2750, 1984
42. Santoro A, Bonadonna G, Bonfante V, et al: Alternating drug combinations in the treatment of advanced Hodgkin's disease. *N Engl J Med* 306:770–775, 1982
43. Straus DJ, Myers J, Passe S, et al: The eight-drug/radiation therapy program (MOPP/ABDV/RT) for advanced Hodgkin's disease. *Cancer* 46:233–240, 1980
44. Gee TS, Yu KP, Clarkson BD: Treatment of adult acute leukemia with arabinosyl cytosine and thioguanine. *Cancer* 23:1019–1032, 1969
45. Crowther D, Bateman CJT, Vartan CP, et al: Combination chemotherapy

using L-asparaginase, daunorubicin, and cytosine arabinoside in adults with acute myelogenous leukaemia. *Br Med J* 4:513–517, 1970

46. Freireich EJ, Keating MJ, Gehan EA, et al: Therapy of acute myelogenous leukemia. *Cancer* 42:874–882, 1978

47. Gunz FW, Vincent PC: Towards a cure of acute granulocytic leukemia? *Leuk Res* 1:51–66, 1977

48. Henderson ES: Treatment of acute leukemia. *Ann Intern Med* 69:628–632, 1968

49. Clarkson BD, Dowling MD, Gee TS, et al: Treatment of acute leukemia in adults. *Cancer* 36:775–795, 1975

50. Crosby WH: To treat or not to treat acute granulocytic leukemia. *Arch Intern Med* 122:79–80, 1968

51. Boggs DR, Wintrobe MM, Cartwright GE: To treat or not to treat acute granulocytic leukemia. *Arch Intern Med* 123:568–570, 1969

52. Crosby WH: Letter to editor. *Arch Intern Med* 123:206–207, 1969

53. Dameshek W: Treatment of acute granulocytic leukemia. *Arch Intern Med* 123:725–726, 1969

54. Lee SL, Rosner F: Letter to editor. *Arch Intern Med* 123:205–206, 1969

55. Keating MJ, McCredie KB, Bodey GP, et al: Improved prospects for long-term survival in adults with acute myelogenous leukemia. *JAMA* 248:2481–2486, 1982

56. Kantarjian HM, Keating MJ, Walters RS: The characteristics and outcome of patients with late relapse acute myelogenous leukemia. *J Clin Oncol* 6:232–238, 1988

57. Keating MJ, Cork A, Broach Y, et al: Toward a clinically relevant classification of acute myelogenous leukemia. *Leuk Res* 11:119–133, 1987

58. Peterson BA, Bloomfield CD: Long-term disease-free survival in acute nonlymphocytic leukemia. *Blood* 57:1144–1147, 1981

59. Pinkel D: History and development of total therapy for acute lymphocytic leukemia. In *Leukemia Research: Advances in Cell Biology and Treatment*, Murphy SB, Gilbert JR (eds.). New York, Elsevier, pp. 189–201, 1982

60. Sullivan MP: Intracranial complications of leukemia in children. *Pediatrics* 20:757–781, 1957

61. Sansone G: Pathomorphosis of acute infantile leukaemia treated with modern therapeutic agents: "Meningoleukaemia" and Frölich's obesity. *Ann Paediatr* 183:33–41, 1954

62. Rieselbach RE, Morse EE, Rall DP, et al: Treatment of meningeal leukemia with intrathecal aminopterin. *Cancer Chemother Rep* 16:191–196, 1962

63. Shaw RK, Moore EW, Freireich EJ, et al: Meningeal leukemia: A syndrome resulting from increased intracranial pressure in patients with acute leukemia. *Neurology* 10:823–833, 1960

64. Editor: Treating the nervous system in acute leukemia. *Lancet* 1:297–298, 1972

65. Kay HEM, Knapton PJ, O'Sullivan JP, et al: Severe neurological damage associated with methotrexate therapy. *Lancet* 2:542, 1971

66. Moore EW, Thomas LB, Shaw RK, et al: The central nervous system in acute leukemia: A postmortem study of 117 consecutive cases with particular reference to hemorrhage, leukemic infiltrations and the syndrome of meningeal leukemia. *Arch Intern Med* 105:451–468, 1960

67. Bleyer WA: Central nervous system leukemia. *Pediatr Clin North Am* 35(4):789–814, 1988

6. Supportive Therapy

1. Feinblatt HM: *Transfusion of Blood*. New York, Macmillan, pp. 1–11, 1926

2. Lower R: *Philos Trans Soc Lond* 1:128, 352, 1665–66

3. Oberman HA: The history of blood transfusion. In *Clinical Practice of Blood Transfusion*, Petz LD, Swisher SN (eds.). New York, Churchill Livingstone, pp. 9–28, 1981

4. Pepys S: *The Diary of Samuel Pepys*, vol. 6, Wheatley H (ed.). London, Bell & Sons, p. 64, 1896

5. Mollison PL: Preface. In *Blood Transfusion in Clinical Medicine*, ed. 7. Oxford, Blackwell Scientific Publications, p. xxi, 1983

6. Denis JP: *Philos Trans Soc Lond* 1:617, 1665–66

7. Tardy MC: Traité de l'écoulement du sang d'un homme dans les veines d'un autre et de ses utilitiz. Doct en Méd. Paris, Bray & Barbin, pp. 1–15

8. Brown H: Jean Denis and transfusion of blood, Paris, 1667–1668. *Isis* 39:15–29, 1948

9. Denis J: *Letter written to M. de Montmor, 25 June, 1667* (adapted). Paris, Cusson, pp. 1–15

10. Denis JP: *Philos Trans Soc Lond* 4:617, 1668

11. Bischoff TLW: Beiträge zur Lehre von dem Blute und der Transfusion desselben. *Arch Anat Physiol Wissensch Med*:347, 1835

12. Smith T: Transfusion of blood in the case of a patient suffering from purpura. *Lancet* 1:837–838, 1873

13. Landsteiner K: Zur Kenntnis der antifermentativen, lytischen und agglutinierenden Wirkungen des Blutserums und der Lymphe. *Zentralbl Bakteriol* 27:357–362, 1900

14. Shattock SG: Chromocyte clumping in acute pneumonia and certain other diseases, and the significance of the buffy coat in the shed blood. *J Pathol Bacteriol* 6:303–314, 1900

15. Janský J: Haematologické studie u psychotiků. *Sb Klin Rabot Terapeuticheskago* 8:35, 1906–7

16. Crile GW: The technic of direct transfusion of blood. *Ann Surg* 46:329–332, 1907

17. Crile GW: *Hemorrhage and Transfusion: An Experimental and Clinical Research*. New York, D. Appleton, 1909.

18. Von Ziemssen: Über die subcutane Blutinjection und über eine einfache Methode der intravenösen Transfusion. *Munch Med Wochenschr* 39:323, 1892

19. Lindeman E: Simple syringe transfusion with special cannulas: A new method applicable to infants and adults. Preliminary report. *Am J Dis Child* 6:28–32, 1913

20. Unger LJ: A new method of syringe transfusion. *JAMA* 64:582–584, 1915

21. Hustin: Principe d'une nouvelle méthode de transfusion muqueuse. *J Med Brux* 12:436, 1914

22. Agote L: Nueve procedimiento para la transfusión del sangre. *Anal Inst Modelo Clin Med Buenos Aires*, (January) 1915

23. Duke WW: The relation of blood platelets to hemorrhagic disease: Description of a method for determining the bleeding time and coagulation time and report of three cases of hemorrhagic disease relieved by transfusion. *JAMA* 55:1185–1192, 1910

24. Cohn EJ: Preface. In *Blood Cells and Plasma Proteins*, Tullis JL (ed.). New York, Academic Press, pp. ix–xii, 1953

25. Cronkite EP, Jackson DP: Use of platelet transfusions in hemorrhagic disease. *Prog Hematol* 2:239–257, 1959

26. Cronkite EP, Jacobs GJ, Brecher G, et al: The hemorrhagic phase of the acute radiation syndrome due to exposure of the whole body to penetrating, ionizing radiation. *Am J Roentgenol* 67:796–803, 1952

27. Dillard GHL, Brecher G, Cronkite EP: Separation, concentration and transfusion of platelets. *Proc Soc Exp Biol Med* 78:796–799, 1951

28. Cronkite EP, Brecher G: Defects in hemostasis produced by whole body irradiation. In *Transactions of the Fifth Conference on Blood Clotting & Allied Problems*. New York, Josiah Macy, Jr. Foundation, pp. 171–212, 1952

29. Brecher G, Cronkite EP: The effects of platelet transfusion in dogs made pancytopenic by x-radiation. *NY State J Med* 53:544–547, 1953

30. Cronkite EP, Brecher G, Wilbur KM: Development and use of a canine blood donor colony for experimental purposes: I. Leucocyte and platelet transfusions in irradiation aplasia of the dog bone marrow. *Milit Surg* 114:359–365, 1954

31. Cronkite EP, Brecher G: The experimental therapy of the hemorrhagic phase of the radiation syndrome with platelet transfusions. *Acta Radiol* 116(Suppl):376–380, 1954

32. Hirsch EO, Favre-Gilly J, Dameshek W: Thrombopathic thrombocytopenia: Successful transfusion of blood platelets. *Blood* 5:568–580, 1950

33. Hirsch EO, Gardner FH: The transfusion of human blood platelets. *J Lab Clin Med* 39:556–569, 1952

34. Brecher G, Schneiderman M, Cronkite EP: Reproducibility and constancy of platelet count. *Am J Clin Pathol* 23:15–26, 1953

35. Gaydos LA, Freireich EJ, Mantel N: The quantitative relation between platelet count and hemorrhage in patients with acute leukemia. *N Engl J Med* 266:905–909, 1962

36. Freireich EJ, Schmidt PJ, Schneiderman MA, et al: A comparative study of the effect of transfusion of fresh and preserved whole blood on bleeding in patients with acute leukemia. *N Engl J Med* 260:6–11, 1959

37. Zubrod CG: Origins and development of chemotherapy research at the National Cancer Institute. *Cancer Treat Rep* 68:9–19, 1984
38. Freireich EJ, Kliman A, Gaydos LA, et al: Response to repeated platelet transfusion from the same donor. *Ann Intern Med* 59:277–287, 1963
39. Djerassi I, Farber S, Evans AE: Transfusions of fresh platelet concentrates to patients with secondary thrombocytopenia. *N Engl J Med* 268:221–226, 1963
40. Alvarado J, Djerassi I, Farber S: Transfusion of fresh concentrated platelets to children with acute leukemia. *J Pediatr* 67:13–22, 1965
41. Menitove JE: Platelet transfusions for alloimmunized patients. *Clin Oncol* 2:587–609, 1983
42. Kelton JG, Ali AM: Platelet transfusions: A critical appraisal. *Clin Oncol* 2:549–585, 1983
43. McCredie KB, Hester JP, Freireich EJ, et al: Platelet and leukocyte transfusions in acute leukemia. *Hum Pathol* 5:699–708, 1974
44. Aster RH, Jandl JH: Platelet sequestration in man. I. Methods. *J Clin Invest* 43:843–855, 1964
45. Murphy S: Platelet storage for transfusion. *Semin Hematol* 22:165–177, 1985
46. Murphy S, Gardner FH: Platelet storage at 22°C.: Role of gas transport across plastic containers in maintenance of viability. *Blood* 46:209–218, 1975
47. Eisenstaedt R: Blood component therapy in the treatment of platelet disorders. *Semin Hematol* 23:1–7, 1986
48. Barton JC, Conrad ME: Beneficial effects of hepatitis in patients with acute myelogenous leukemia. *Ann Intern Med* 90:188–190, 1979
49. Foon KA, Yale C, Clodfelter K, et al: Post-transfusion hepatitis in acute myelogenous leukemia: Effect on survival. *JAMA* 244:1806–1807, 1980
50. McCredie KB, Freireich EJ: Blood component therapy. In *Cancer Medicine*, Holland JF, Frei E III (eds.). Philadelphia, Lea & Febiger, pp. 1115–1129, 1973
51. Strumia MM: Effect of leukocyte cream injections in the treatment of neutropenias. *Am J Med Sci* 187:527–544, 1934
52. Vallejos C, McCredie KB, Bodey GP, et al: White blood cell transfusions for control of infections in neutropenic patients. *Transfusion* 15:28–33, 1975
53. Graw RG, Goldstein IM, Eyre HJ, et al: Histocompatibility testing for leukocyte transfusions. *Lancet* 2:77–78, 1970
54. Winston DJ, Ho WG, Howell CL, et al: Cytomegalovirus infections associated with leukocyte transfusions. *Ann Intern Med* 93:671–675, 1980
55. Schiffer CA: Principles of granulocyte transfusion therapy. *Med Clin North Am* 61:1119–1131, 1977
56. Schimpff SC, Gaya H, Klastersky J, et al: Three antibiotic regimens in the treatment of infection in febrile granulocytopenic patients with cancer: The EORTC international antimicrobial therapy project group. *J Infect Dis* 137:14–29, 1978

57. Bodey GP: Infection in cancer patients. *Am J Med* 81(Suppl 1A):11–26, 1986

58. Bodey GP: Infections in patients with cancer. In *Cancer Medicine*, Holland JF, Frei E III (eds). Philadelphia, Lea & Febiger, pp. 1339–1372, 1982

59. Bodey GP, Nies BA, Mohberg NR, et al: Use of gamma globulin in infection in acute leukemia patients. *JAMA* 190:1099–1106, 1964

60. Bodey GP, Nies BA, Mohberg NR, et al: The effect of adrenal corticosteroid therapy on infections in acute leukemia. *Am J Med Sci* 250:162–167, 1965

61. Bodey GP, Jadeja L, Elting L: *Pseudomonas* bacteremia: Retrospective analysis of 410 episodes. *Arch Intern Med* 145:1621–1629, 1985

62. Fainstein V, Bodey GP: Single-agent therapy for infections in neutropenic cancer patients. *Am J Med* 79(Suppl 2A):83–88, 1985

63. Bodey GP, Rodriguez V, Luce JK: Carbenicillin therapy of gram-negative bacilli infections. *Am J Med Sci* 257:408–414, 1969

64. Bodey GP, Whitecar JP, Middlemann E, et al: Carbenicillin therapy for pseudomonal infections. *JAMA* 218:61–66, 1971

65. Klastersky J, Cappel R, Daneau D: Therapy with carbenicillin and gentamicin for patients with cancer and severe infections caused by gram-negative rods. *Cancer* 31:331–336, 1973

66. Rodriguez VK, Bodey GP, Horikoshi N, et al: Ticarcillin therapy of infections. *Antimicrob Agents Chemother* 4:427–431, 1973

67. Hersh EM, Bodey GP, Nies BA, et al: Causes of death in acute leukemia. *JAMA* 193:105–109, 1965

68. Pizzo PA, Thaler M, Hathorn J, et al: New beta-lactam antibiotics in granulocytopenic patients: New options and new questions. *Am J Med* 79(Suppl 2A):75–82, 1985

69. Bodey GP, Rodriguez V, Chang HY, et al: Fever and infection in leukemic patients: A study of 494 consecutive patients. *Cancer* 41:1610–1622, 1978

70. Pizzo PA, Ladisch SL, Gill F, et al: Increasing incidence of gram-positive sepsis in cancer patients. *Med Pediatr Oncol* 5:241–244, 1978

71. Bodey GP, Buckley M, Sathe YS, et al: Quantitative relationships between circulating leukocytes and infection in patients with acute leukemia. *Ann Intern Med* 64:328–340, 1966

72. Bodey GP, Nies BA, Freireich EJ: Multiple organism septicemia in acute leukemia: Analysis of 54 episodes. *Arch Intern Med* 116:266–272, 1965

73. Craig JM, Farber S: The development of disseminated visceral mycosis during therapy for acute leukemia (abstract). *Am J Pathol* 29:601, 1953

74. Baker RD: Leukopenia and therapy in leukemia as factors predisposing to fatal mycoses: Mucormycosis, aspergillosis, and cryptococcosis. *Am J Clin Pathol* 37:358–363, 1962

75. Bodey GP: Fungal infection and fever of unknown origin in neutropenic patients. *Am J Med* 80(Suppl 5C):112–119, 1986

76. Estey EH, Keating MJ, McCredie KB, et al: Causes of initial remission induction failure in acute myelogenous leukemia. *Blood* 60:309–315, 1982

77. Louria DB, Stiff DP, Bennett B: Disseminated moniliasis in the adult. *Medicine (Baltimore)* 41:307–333, 1962

78. Maksymiuk AW, Thongprasert S, Hopfer R, et al: Systemic candidiasis in cancer patients. *Am J Med* 77(Suppl 4D):20–27, 1984

79. Meunier F: Prevention of mycoses in immunocompromised patients. *Rev Infect Dis* 9:408–416, 1987

80. Lopez-Berestein G, Fainstein V, Hopfer R, et al: Liposomal amphotericin B for the treatment of systemic fungal infections in patients with cancer. *J Infect Dis* 151:704–710, 1985

81. Meunier F, Klastersky J: Recent developments in prophylaxis and therapy of invasive fungal infections in granulocytopenic cancer patients. *Eur J Cancer Clin Oncol* 24:539–544, 1988

82. Meyers JD: Infection in bone marrow transplant recipients. *Am J Med* 81(Suppl 1A):27–38, 1986

83. Peterson PK, Ramsay NKC, Rhame F, et al: A prospective study of infectious diseases following bone marrow transplantation. *Infect Control* 4:81–89, 1983

84. Winston DJ, Ho WG, Champlin RE, et al: Infectious complications of bone marrow transplantation. *Exp Hematol* 12:205–215, 1984

85. Reyniers JA, Trexler PC, Scruggs W, et al: Observations on germ-free and conventional albino rats after total-body x-irradiation (abstract). *Radiat Res* 5:591, 1956

86. Wilson BR: Survival studies of whole-body x-irradiated germ-free (axenic) mice. *Radiat Res* 20:477–483, 1963

87. White LP, Claflin EF: Nitrogen mustard: Diminution of toxicity in axenic mice. *Science* 140:1400–1401, 1963

88. Bodey GP, Rosenbaum B: Effect of prophylactic measures on the microbial flora of patients in protected environment units. *Medicine (Baltimore)* 53:209–228, 1974

89. Bodey GP, Freireich EJ, Frei E III: Studies of patients in a laminar air flow unit. *Cancer* 24:972–980, 1969

90. Bodey GP, Gehan EA, Freireich EJ, et al: Protected environment-prophylactic antibiotic program in the chemotherapy of acute leukemia. *Am J Med Sci* 262:138–151, 1971

91. Levine AS, Siegel SE, Schreiber AD, et al: Protected environments and prophylactic antibiotics: A prospective controlled study of their utility in the therapy of acute leukemia. *N Engl J Med* 288:477–483, 1973

92. Bodey GP, Rodriguez V, Cabanillas F, et al: Protected environment-prophylactic antibiotic program for malignant lymphoma: Randomized trial during chemotherapy to induce remission. *Am J Med* 66:74–81, 1979

93. Bodey GP, Rodriguez V, Murphy WK, et al: Protected environment-prophylactic antibiotic program for malignant sarcomas: Randomized trial during remission induction chemotherapy. *Cancer* 47:2422–2429, 1981

94. Hortobagyi GN, Buzdar AU, Bodey GP, et al: High-dose induction chemotherapy of metastatic breast cancer in protected environment: A prospective randomized study. *J Clin Oncol* 5:178–184, 1987

95. Bodey GP: Symposium on infectious complications of neoplastic disease (part II): Current status of prophylaxis of infection with protected environments. *Am J Med* 76:678–684, 1984

96. Armstrong D: Symposium on infectious complications of neoplastic disease (part II): Protected environments are discomforting and expensive and do not offer meaningful protection. *Am J Med* 76:685–689, 1984

97. Mitchell CD: Management of infections in the neutropenic child with cancer. *Pediatr Ann* 17:677–686, 1988

98. Osgood EE, Muscovitz AN: Culture of human bone marrow. *JAMA* 106:1888–1890, 1936

99. Osgood EE: The histogenesis, classification and identification of the cells of the blood and marrow based on cultures and hematologic studies of human marrow and blood. *Am J Clin Pathol* 8:59–73, 1938

100. Osgood EE, Riddle MC, Mathews TJ: Aplastic anemia treated with daily transfusions and intravenous marrow: Case report. *Ann Intern Med* 13:357–367, 1939

101. Morrison M, Samwick AA: Intramedullary (sternal) transfusion of human bone marrow. *JAMA* 115:1708–1711, 1940

102. Bortin MM: A compendium of reported human bone marrow transplants. *Transplantation* 9:571–587, 1970

103. Lorenz E, Uphoff D, Reid TR, et al: Modification of irradiation injury in mice and guinea pigs by bone marrow injections. *JNCI* 12:197–201, 1951

104. Rekers PE: Transplantation of bone marrow into dogs that have received total body single dose radiation. University of Rochester Atomic Energy Project, No. 11, 1948

105. Thomas ED, Lochte HL Jr, Lu WC, et al: Intravenous infusion of bone marrow in patients receiving radiation and chemotherapy. *N Engl J Med* 257:491–496, 1957

106. Mathé G, Jammet H, Pendic B, et al: Transfusions et greffes de moelle osseuse homologue chez des humains irradiés à haute dose accidentellement. *Rev Fr Etudes Clin Biol* 4:226–238, 1959

107. Gordon-Smith EC: Bone marrow transplantation for aplastic anemia and leukaemia. *Triangle* 17:63–73, 1978

108. Bach FH: Bone-marrow transplantation in a patient with the Wiskott-Aldrich syndrome. *Lancet* 2:1364–1366, 1968

109. Gatti RA, Allen HD, Meuwissen HJ: Immunological reconstitution of sex-linked lymphopenic immunological deficiency. *Lancet* 2:1366–1369, 1968

110. DeKoning J, Van Bekkum DW, Dicke KA: Transplantation of bone-marrow cells and fetal thymus in an infant with lymphopenic immunological deficiency. *Lancet* 1:1223–1227, 1969

111. Thomas ED, Storb R, Clift RA, et al: Bone marrow transplantation: Part 2. *N Engl J Med* 292:895–902, 1975

112. Santos GW: Immunosuppression for clinical marrow transplantation. *Semin Hematol* 11:341–351, 1974

113. Thomas ED, Storb R, Clift RA, et al: Bone marrow transplantation: Part 1. *N Engl J Med* 292:832–843, 1975

114. Thomas ED, Buckner CD, Banaji M, et al: One hundred patients with acute leukemia treated with chemotherapy, total body irradiation and allogeneic marrow transplantation. *Blood* 49:511–533, 1977

115. Zwaan FE, Jansen J: Bone marrow transplantation in acute nonlymphoblastic leukemia. *Semin Hematol* 21:36–42, 1984

116. Thomas ED, Buckner CD, Clift RA, et al: Marrow transplantation for patients with acute nonlymphoblastic leukemia in first remission. *N Engl J Med* 301:597–599, 1979

117. Appelbaum FR, Dahlberg S, Thomas ED, et al: Bone marrow transplantation or chemotherapy after remission induction for adults with acute nonlymphoblastic leukemia: A prospective comparison. *Ann Intern Med* 101:581–588, 1984

118. Zander AR, Keating M, Dicke K, et al: A comparison of marrow transplantation with chemotherapy for adults with acute leukemia of poor prognosis in first complete remission. *J Clin Oncol* 6:1548–1557, 1988

119. Champlin RE, Ho WG, Gale RP, et al: Treatment of acute myelogenous leukemia: A prospective controlled trial of bone marrow transplantation versus consolidation chemotherapy. *Ann Intern Med* 102:285–291, 1985

120. Buckner CD, Clift RA, Fefer A, et al: Treatment of blastic transformation of chronic granulocytic leukemia by high dose cyclophosphamide, total body irradiation and infusion of cryopreserved autologous marrow. *Exp Hematol* 2:138–146, 1974

121. Minot GR, Buckman TE, Isaacs R: Chronic myelogenous leukemia: Age, incidence, duration and benefit derived from irradiation. *JAMA* 82:1489–1494, 1924

122. Fefer A, Clift RA, Thomas ED: Allogeneic marrow transplantation for chronic granulocytic leukemia. *JNCI* 76:1295–1299, 1986

123. Fefer A, Cheever MA, Greenberg PD: Identical twin (syngeneic) marrow transplantation for hematologic cancers. *JNCI* 76:1269–1273, 1986

124. Speck B, Bortin MM, Champlin R, et al: Allogeneic bone marrow transplantation for chronic myelogenous leukemia. *Lancet* 1:665–668, 1984

125. Speck B: Bone marrow transplantation. *Acta Haematol* 72:145–154, 1984

126. Klingemann HG, Storb R, Fefer A, et al: Bone marrow transplantation in patients aged 45 years and older. *Blood* 67:770–776, 1986

127. Barnes DWH, Corp MJ, Loutit JF, et al: Treatment of murine leukaemia with x-rays and homologous bone marrow. *Br Med J* 2:626–627, 1956

128. Fefer A, Sullivan KM, Weiden P, et al: Graft versus leukemia effect in man: The relapse rate of acute leukemia is lower after allogeneic than after syngeneic marrow transplantation. *Prog Clin Biol Res* 244:401–408, 1986

129. Mathé G, Amiel JL, Schwarzenberg L, et al: Adoptive immunotherapy of acute leukemia: Experimental and clinical results. *Cancer Res* 25:1525–1531, 1965

130. Weiden PL, Flournoy N, Thomas ED, et al: Antileukemic effect of graft-

versus-host disease in human recipients of allogeneic-marrow grafts. *N Engl J Med* 300:1068–1073, 1979

131. Gale RP, Champlin RE: How does bone marrow transplantation cure leukemia? *Lancet* 2:28–29, 1984

132. Butturini A, Bortin MM, Seeger RC, et al: Graft-vs-leukemia following bone marrow transplantation: A model of immunotherapy in man. *Prog Clin Biol Res* 244: 371–390, 1986

133. Gale RP, Bortin MM: Bone marrow transplantation in leukemia: International Bone Marrow Transplant Registry (IBMTR) data. *Int J Cell Cloning* 3:236–237, 1985

134. Kurnick NB, Montano A, Gerdes JC, et al: Preliminary observations in the treatment of postirradiation hematopoietic depression in man by the infusion of stored autogenous bone marrow. *Ann Intern Med* 49:973–986, 1958

135. McGovern JJ Jr, Russell PS, Atkins L, et al: Treatment of terminal leukemic relapse by total-body irradiation and intravenous infusion of stored autologous bone marrow obtained during remission. *N Engl J Med* 260:675–683, 1959

136. Dicke KA, Spitzer G, Peters L, et al: Autologous bone-marrow transplantation in relapsed adult acute leukemia. *Lancet* 1:514–517, 1979

137. Horwitz LJ, Dicke KA, Jagannath S, et al: Perspectives in treatment of adult leukemia with high dose cytoreductive therapy and autologous bone marrow treated ex vivo. In *Recent Advances and Future Directions in Bone Marrow Transplantation*, Baum SJ, Santos GW, Takaku F (eds.). New York, Springer-Verlag, pp. 58–73, 1987

138. Santos GW, Colvin OM: Pharmacological purging of bone marrow with reference to autografting. *Clin Haematol* 15:67–83, 1986

139. Dicke KA, Jagannath S, Walters RS, et al: The role of autologous bone marrow transplantation in acute leukemia. *Ann NY Acad Sci* 511:468–472, 1987

140. Bortin MM, Rimm AA: Increasing utilization of bone marrow transplantation. *Transplantation* 42:229–234, 1986

7. Biologic Response Modifiers

1. Coley WB: Contributions to the knowledge of sarcoma. *Ann Surg* 14:199–220, 1891

2. Goldstein D, Laszlo J: The role of interferon in cancer therapy: A current perspective. *CA* 38:258–277, 1988

3. Oldham RK: Why another journal? (editorial). *J Biol Response Mod* 1:1–2, 1982

4. Oldham RK: Biological response modifiers program. *J Biol Response Mod* 1:81–100, 1982

5. Gutterman J: Overview of advances in the use of biological proteins in human cancer. *Semin Oncol* 5(Suppl 5):2–6, 1988

6. Hawkins MJ, Hoth DF, Wittes RE: Clinical development of biological response modifiers: Comparison with cytotoxic drugs. *Semin Oncol* 13:132–140, 1986

7. DeVita VT Jr: Principles of chemotherapy. In *Cancer: Principles and Practice of Oncology*, DeVita VT Jr, Hellman S, Rosenberg SA (eds.). Philadelphia, Lippincott, pp. 144–145, 1982

8. Shoemaker RH, Wolpert-DeFilippes MK, Kern DH, et al: Application of a human tumor colony-forming assay to new drug screening. *Cancer Res* 45:2145–2153, 1985

9. Fidler IJ, Berendt M, Oldham RK: Rationale for and design of a screening procedure for the assessment of biological response modifiers for cancer treatment. *J Biol Response Mod* 1:15–26, 1982

10. Talmadge JE, Herberman RB: The preclinical screening laboratory: Evaluation of immunomodulatory and therapeutic properties of biological response modifiers. *Cancer Treat Rep* 70:171–182, 1986

11. Crispen RG: BCG vaccine in perspective. *Semin Oncol* 1:311–317, 1974

12. Gunby P: Answer is still out regarding BCG's possible anticancer role. *JAMA* 248:2209–2210, 1982

13. Holmgren I: La tuberculine et le BCG chez les cancereux. *Schweiz Med Wochenschr* 65:1203–1206, 1935

14. Halpern BN, Biozzi G, Stiffel C, et al: Effet de la stimulation du système réticulo-endothélial par l'inoculation du bacille de Calmette-Guérin sur le développement d'épithélioma atypique T–8 de Guérin chez le rat. *C R Soc Biol (Paris)* 153:919–923, 1959

15. Powles RL, Crowther D, Bateman CJT: Immunotherapy for acute myelogenous leukaemia. *Br J Cancer* 28:365–376, 1973

16. Old LJ, Clarke DA, Benacerraf B, et al: Effect of bacillus Calmette-Guérin infection on transplanted tumours in the mouse. *Nature* 184:291–292, 1959

17. Old LJ, Clarke DA, Benacerraf B, et al: The reticulo-endothelial system and the neoplastic process. *Ann NY Acad Sci* 88:264–280, 1960

18. Ambrosch F, Wiedermann G, Krepler P: Studies on the influence of BCG vaccination on infantile leukemia. *Dev Biol Stand* 58(part A):419–424, 1986

19. Härö AS: The effect of BCG vaccination and tuberculosis on the risk of leukaemia. *Dev Biol Stand* 58(part A):433–449, 1986

20. Villasor RP: The clinical use of BCG vaccine in stimulating host resistance to cancer: II. Immunochemotherapy in advanced cancer. *J Philippine Med Assoc* 41:619–632, 1965.

21. Mathé G, Amiel JL, Schwarzenberg L, et al: Active immunotherapy for acute lymphoblastic leukemia. *Lancet* 1:697–699, 1969

22. Davignon L, Robillard P, Lemonde P, et al: B.C.G. vaccination and leukaemia mortality. *Lancet* 2:638, 1970

23. Leukemia Committee and the Working Party on Leukemia in Childhood: Treatment of acute lymphoblastic leukemia: Comparison of immunotherapy (BCG), intermittent methotrexate, and no therapy after a five-month intensive cytotoxic regimen (Concord Trial). *Br Med J* 4:189–194, 1971

24. Gutterman JU, Rodriguez V, Mavligit G, et al: Chemoimmunotherapy of adult acute leukemia: Prolongation of remission in myeloblastic leukaemia with B.C.G. *Lancet* 2:1405–1409, 1974

25. Carswell EA, Old LJ, Kassel RL, et al: An endotoxin-induced serum factor that causes necrosis of tumors. Proc Natl Acad Sci USA 72:3666–3670, 1975

26. Cachran AJ, Buyse ME, Lejeune FJ, et al: Adjuvant reactivity predicts survival in patients with "high risk" primary malignant melanoma treated with systemic BCG. *Int J Cancer* 28:543–550, 1981

27. Hortobagyi GN, Buzdar AU, Blumenschein GR, et al: Prediction of survival by degree of reactivity to BCG in patients with metastatic breast cancer. *Dev Biol Stand* 58(part A):357–363, 1986

28. DeVita VT Jr: Summary. Proceedings of the International Symposium on Leukemia Cell Biology and Therapy, Memphis, TN, May 19–22, 1982. In *Leukemia Research: Advances in Cell Biology and Treatment*, Murphy SB, Gilbert JR (eds.). New York, Elsevier, pp. 295–305, 1982

29. Shorter E: *The Health Century.* New York, Doubleday, pp. 234–259, 1987

30. Isaacs A, Lindenmann JJ: Virus interference: The interferon. *Proc R Soc Lond [Biol]* 147:258–267, 1957

31. Kirkwood JM, Ernstoff MS: Interferons in the treatment of human cancer. *J Clin Oncol* 2:336–352, 1984

32. Working Party on Human Interferon: Progress towards trials of human interferon in man. *Ann NY Acad Sci* 173:770–781, 1970

33. Atanasiu P, Chany C: Action d'un interféron provenant de cellules malignes sur l'infection expérimentale du hamster nouveau-né par le virus du polyome. *C R Acad Sci [III]* 251:1687–1689, 1960

34. Gresser I: Antitumor effects of interferon. *Adv Cancer Res* 16:97–140, 1972

35. Allison AC: Interference with, and interferon production by, polyoma virus. *Virology* 15:47–61, 1961

36. Strander H, Cantell K, Carlström G, et al: Clinical and laboratory investigations on man: Systemic administration of potent interferon to man. *JNCI* 51:733–742, 1973

37. Sehgal PB: The interferon gene. *Biochem Biophys Acta* 695:17–33, 1982

38. Toufexis A: The big IF in cancer. *Time*, pp. 60–66, March 31, 1980

39. Falcoff E, Falcoff R, Fournier F, et al: Production en masse, purification partielle et caractérisation d'un interféron destive à des essais thérapeutiques humains. *Ann Immunol (Paris)* 3:562–569, 1966

40. Strander H, Cantell K: Studies on antiviral and antitumor effects of human leukocyte interferon in vitro and in vivo. In *The Production and Use of Interferon for the Treatment and Prevention of Human Virus Infections*, In Vitro Monograph No. 3, Waymouth C (ed.). Rockville, MD, Tissue Culture Association, pp. 49–56, 1974

41. Diamandopoulos GT: Leukemia, lymphoma, and osteosarcoma induced in the Syrian golden hamster by Simian virus 40. *Science* 176:173–175, 1972

42. Strander H, Cantell K, Ingimarson S, et al: Interferon treatment of osteogenic sarcoma: A clinical trial. In *Conference on Modulation of Host Immune Resistance in the Prevention or Treatment of Induced Neo-*

plasias, vol. 28, Chirigos M (ed.). Washington, DC, U.S. Government Printing Office, pp. 377–381, 1974

43. Hill NO, Pardue A, Kahn A, et al: High-dose human leukocyte interferon trials in leukemia and cancer. *Med Pediatr Oncol* 9:82, 1981
44. Gutterman JU, Fine S, Quesada J, et al: Recombinant leukocyte A interferon: Pharmacokinetics, single-dose tolerance, and biologic effects in cancer patients. *Ann Intern Med* 96:549–556, 1982
45. Hersh EM, Quesada J, Keating MJ: Host defense factors and prognosis in hairy cell leukemia. *Leuk Res* 6:625–637, 1982
46. Stewart DJ, Smith TL, Keating MJ, et al: Prognostic factors in hairy cell leukemia. *Cancer* 53:1198–1201, 1984
47. Quesada JR, Reuben J, Manning JT, et al: Alpha interferon for induction of remission in hairy-cell leukemia. *N Engl J Med* 310:15–18, 1984
48. Quesada JR, Hersh EM, Manning J, et al: Treatment of hairy cell leukemia with recombinant α-interferon. *Blood* 68:493–497, 1986
49. Loddeke L: Interferon's effectiveness expands: Drugs work against 10 forms of cancer. *Houston Post*, p. 6E, June 27, 1988
50. Spiers ASD, Parekh SJ, Bishop MB: Hairy-cell leukemia: Induction of complete remission with pentostatin (2'-deoxycoformycin). *J Clin Oncol* 2:1336–1342, 1984
51. Golomb HM, Ratain MJ, Moormeier J: What is the choice of treatment for hairy cell leukemia? *J Clin Oncol* 7:156–158, 1989
52. Cheson BD, Martin A: Clinical trials in hairy cell leukemia: Current status and future directions. *Ann Intern Med* 106:871–878, 1987
53. Talpaz M, McCredie KB, Mavligit GM, et al: Leukocyte interferon-induced myeloid cytoreduction in chronic myelogenous leukemia. *Blood* 62:689–692, 1983
54. Talpaz M, Kantarjian HM, McCredie K, et al: Hematologic remission and cytogenetic improvement induced by recombinant human interferon alpha in chronic myelogenous leukemia. *N Engl J Med* 314:1065–1069, 1986
55. Talpaz M, Kantarjian HM, McCredie KB, et al: Clinical investigation of human alpha interferon in chronic myelogenous leukemia. *Blood* 69:1280–1288, 1987
56. Kurzrock R, Talpaz M, Kantarjian H, et al: Therapy of chronic myelogenous leukemia with recombinant interferon-γ. *Blood* 70:943–947, 1987
57. Morgan DA, Ruscetti FW, Gallo RC: Selective in vitro growth of T-lymphocytes from normal human bone marrow. *Science* 193:1007–1008, 1976
58. Merz B: Antitumor strategies based on enhancing—and blocking—effects of interleukin-2. *JAMA* 256:1241, 1244, 1986
59. Lifson J, Raubitschek A, Benike C, et al: Purified interleukin-2 induces proliferation of fresh human lymphocytes in the absence of exogenous stimuli. *J Biol Response Mod* 5:61–72, 1986
60. Hammer SM, Gillis JM: Effects of recombinant interleukin-2 on resting human T lymphocytes. *J Biol Response Mod* 5:36–44, 1986
61. Rosenberg SA, Grimm EA, McGrogan M, et al: Biological activity of

recombinant human interleukin-2 produced in *Escherichia coli*. *Science* 223:1412–1415, 1984

62. Taniguchi T, Matsui H, Fujita T, et al: Structure and expression of a cloned cDNA for human interleukin-2. *Nature* 302:305–310, 1983

63. Seigel LJ, Harper ME, Wong-Staal F, et al: Gene for T-cell growth factor: Location on human chromosome 4q and feline chromosome B1. *Science* 223:175–178, 1984

64. Kolitz JE, Welte K, Sykora KW, et al: Interleukin 2: A review. *Arznei-mittelforschung* 35:1607–1615, 1985

65. Lotze MT, Grimm EA, Mazumder A, et al: Lysis of fresh and cultured autologous tumor by human lymphocytes cultured in T-cell growth factor. *Cancer Res* 41:4420–4425, 1981

66. Rosenberg SA, Lotze MT, Muul LM, et al: Observations on the systemic administration of autologous lymphokine-activated killer cells and re-combinant interleukin-2 to patients with metastatic cancer. *N Engl J Med* 313:1485–1492, 1985

67. Lotze MT, Chang AE, Seipp CA, et al: High-dose recombinant interleu-kin-2 in the treatment of patients with disseminated cancer: Responses, treatment-related morbidity, and histologic findings. *JAMA* 256:3117–3124, 1986

68. Moertel CG: On lymphokines, cytokines, and breakthroughs. *JAMA* 256:3141, 1986

69. Boffey PM: The new era in cancer treatment. *Houston Chronicle*, Zest, p. 8, December 4, 1988

70. Pui CH, Ip SH, Kung P, et al: High serum interleukin-2 receptor levels are related to advanced disease and a poor outcome in childhood non-Hodgkin's lymphoma. *Blood* 70:624–628, 1987

71. Jermy A, Lilleyman JS, Jennings R, et al: Spontaneous natural killer cell activity in childhood acute lymphoblastic leukemia. *Eur J Cancer Clin Oncol* 23:1365–1370, 1987

72. Jermy A, Jennings R, Lilleyman JS, et al: Immunomodulation of natural killer activity in children with acute lymphoblastic leukaemia. *Eur J Cancer Clin Oncol* 23:1371–1377, 1987

73. Allison MA, Jones SE, McGuffey P: Phase II trial of outpatient inter-leukin-2 in malignant lymphoma, chronic lymphocytic leukemia, and selected solid tumors. *J Clin Oncol* 7:75–80, 1989

74. Herberman RB: Interleukin-2 therapy of human cancer: Potential ben-efits versus toxicity. *J Clin Oncol* 7:1–4, 1989

75. Hadden JW: Recent advances in the preclinical and clinical immuno-pharmacology of interleukin-2: Emphasis on IL-2 as an immunore-storative agent. *Cancer Detect Prev* 12:537–552, 1988

76. Grimm EA, Mazumder A, Zhang HZ, et al: Lymphokine activated killer cell phenomenon: Lysis of natural killer resistant fresh solid tumor cells by interleukin 2-activated autologous human peripheral blood lympho-cytes. *J Exp Med* 155:823–830, 1982

77. Rosenstein M, Yron I, Kaufmann Y, et al: Lymphokine activated killer cells: Lysis of fresh syngeneic NK-resistant murine tumor cells by lym-phocytes cultured in interleukin-2. *Cancer Res* 44:1946–1953, 1984

78. Lotzová E, Herberman RB: Reassessment of LAK phenomenology: A review. *Nat Immun Cell Growth Regul* 6:109–115, 1987

79. Metschnikoff E: About a yeast infection of *Daphnia*: A contribution to the study about the fighting of phagocytes against organisms that cause disease. *Virchows Arch Pathol Anat Physiol Clin Med* 96:177–195, 1884

80. Morstyn G, Burgess AW: Hemopoietic growth factors: A review. *Cancer Res* 48:5624–5637, 1988

81. Wright AE, Douglas SR: An experimental investigation of the role of the blood fluids in connection with phagocytosis. *Proc R Soc Lond [Biol]* 72:357–370, 1903

82. Carnot P, Deflandre G: Sur l'activité hémopoietique du serum au cours de la régénération du sang. *C R Acad Sci* 143:384–386, 1906

83. Metcalf D: Colony stimulating factors. In *Tissue Growth Factors*, Baserga R (ed.). Berlin, Springer-Verlag, pp. 343–384, 1981

84. Till JE, McCulloch EA: A direct measurement of the radiation sensitivity of normal mouse bone marrow cells. *Radiat Res* 14:213–222, 1961

85. Wolf NS, Trentin JJ: Hemopoietic colony studies: V. Effect of hemopoietic organ stroma on differentiation of pluripotent stem cells. *J Exp Med* 127:205–214, 1968

86. Becker AJ, McCulloch EA, Till JE: Cytological demonstration of the clonal nature of spleen colonies derived from transplanted mouse marrow cells. *Nature* 197:452–454, 1963

87. Pluznik DH, Sachs L: The cloning of normal "mast" cells in tissue culture. *J Cell Physiol* 66:319–324, 1965

88. Wing EJ, Shadduck RK: Colony-stimulating factor. In *Biological Response Modifiers: New Approaches to Disease Intervention*, Torrence PF (ed.). New York, Academic Press, pp. 219–243, 1985

89. Metcalf D, Moore MAS: Regulation of growth and differentiation in haemopoietic colonies growing in agar. In *Proceedings of Ciba Foundation Symposium, London, July 13–14, 1972*. Published as *Haemopoietic Stem Cells*. Amsterdam, Elsevier, pp. 157–175, 1972

90. Quesenberry P, Levitt L: Hematopoietic stem cells. *N Engl J Med* 301:755–760, 819–823, 868–872, 1979

91. Yoffey JM: The LT compartment. In *Proceedings of Ciba Foundation Symposium, London, July 13–14, 1972*. Published as *Haemopoietic Stem Cells*. Amsterdam, Elsevier, pp. 5–39, 1972

92. Stephenson JR, Axelrad AA, McLeod DL, et al: Induction of colonies of hemoglobin-synthesizing cells by erythropoietin in vitro. *Proc Natl Acad Sci USA* 68:1542–1546, 1971

93. Miyajima A, Yokota T, Otsuka T, et al: Interleukins 3 and 4. In *Biological Response Modifiers and Cancer Therapy*, Chiao JW (ed.). New York, Marcel Dekker, pp. 103–148, 1988

94. Glaspy JA, Golde DW: Clinical applications of the myeloid growth factors. *Semin Hematol* 26(Suppl 2):14–17, 1989

95. Chiao JW, Lutton J: Differentiation and maturation inducer factors for leukemia cells. In *Biological Response Modifiers and Cancer Therapy*, Chiao JW (ed.). New York, Marcel Dekker, pp. 363–394, 1988

96. Stanley ER, Metcalf D: Partial purification and some properties of the

factor in normal and leukaemic human urine stimulating mouse bone marrow colony growth in vitro. *Aust J Exp Biol Med Sci* 47:467–483, 1969

97. Sokal G, Michaux JL, van den Berghe H, et al: A new hematopoietic syndrome with a distinct karyotype: The 5q chromosome. *Blood* 46:519–533, 1975

98. Cantrell MA, Anderson D, Cerretti DP, et al: Cloning, sequence, and expression of a human granulocyte/macrophage colony-stimulating factor. *Proc Natl Acad Sci USA* 82:6250–6254, 1985

99. Wong GG, Witek JS, Temple PA, et al: Human GM-CSF: Molecular cloning of the complementary DNA and purification of the natural and recombinant proteins. *Science* 228:810–815, 1985

100. Moore MA: Biologicals for cancer treatment: Growth and differentiating agents. *Hosp Pract* 21:69–80, 1986

101. Friend C, Scher W, Holland JG, et al: Hemoglobin synthesis in murine virus-induced leukemic cells in vitro: Stimulation of erythroid differentiation by dimethyl sulfoxide. *Proc Natl Acad Sci USA* 68:378–382, 1971

102. Abe E, Miyaura C, Sakagami H, et al: Differentiation of mouse myeloid leukemia cells induced by 1 alpha, 25-dihydroxyvitamin D_3. *Proc Natl Acad Sci USA* 78:4990–4994, 1981

103. Gerhartz HH, Wilmanns W: Myeloid progenitors in acute non-lymphocytic leukemia: Prognostic value in remission. *Eur J Cancer Clin Oncol* 22:135–140, 1986

104. Vadhan-Raj S, Keating M, LeMaistre A, et al: Effects of recombinant human granulocyte-macrophage colony-stimulating factor in patients with myelodysplastic syndromes. *N Engl J Med* 317:1545–1552, 1987

105. Vadhan-Raj S, Buescher S, Broxmeyer HE, et al: Stimulation of myelopoiesis in patients with aplastic anemia by recombinant human granulocyte-macrophage colony-stimulating factor. *N Engl J Med* 319:1628–1634, 1988

106. Cosman D: Colony-stimulating factors in vivo and in vitro. *Immunol Today* 9:97–98, 1988

107. Groopman JE: Colony-stimulating factors: Present status and future applications. *Semin Hematol* 25(Suppl 3):30–37, 1988

108. Socinski MA, Cannistra SA, Elias A, et al: Granulocyte-macrophage colony stimulating factor expands the circulating progenitor cell compartment in man. *Lancet* 1:1194–1198, 1988

109. Gabrilove JL: Introduction and overview of hematopoietic growth factors. *Semin Hematol* 26(Suppl 2):1–4, 1989

110. Herberman RB: Cancer therapy by biological response modifiers. *Clin Physiol Biochem* 5:238–248, 1987

8. Human Cytogenetics

1. Waldeyer W: Über Karyokinese und ihre Beziehungen zu den Befruchtungsvorgängen. *Arch Mikroskop Anat Entwicklungsmechanik* 32:1–122, 1888
2. Waldeyer W: On karyokinesis and its relation to the process of fertilization. *Q J Microscop Sci* 30:159–281, 1889
3. Sandberg AA: *The Chromosomes in Human Cancer and Leukemia.* New York, Elsevier North Holland, pp. 1–21, 1980
4. Hecht F: On the origins of cancer genetics and cytogenetics. *Cancer Genet Cytogenet* 29:187–190, 1987
5. Arnold J: Über feinere Struktur der Zellen unter normalen und pathologischen Bedingungen. *Virchows Arch Pathol Anat Physiol Clin Med* 77:181–206, 1879
6. Flemming W: Beitrage zur Kenntniss der Zelle und ihrer Lebenserscheinungen. *Arch Mikroskop Anat Entwicklungsmechanik* 20:1–86, 1882
7. Makino S: *Human Chromosomes.* Amsterdam, North-Holland, pp. 7–21, 1975
8. Flemming W: Über die Chromosomenzahl beim Menschen. *Anat Anz* 14:171–174, 1889
9. Kottler MJ: From 48 to 46: Cytological technique, preconception, and the counting of human chromosomes. *Bull Hist Med* 48:465–502, 1974
10. Baker J: *Cytological Technique.* London, Methuen, 1950
11. Winiwarter H von: Recherches sur l'ovogenèse et l'organogenèse de l'ovaire des mammifères (lapin et homme). *Arch Biol* 17:105–107, 1900
12. Winiwarter H von: Études sur la spermatogenèse humaine. (I. Cellules de Sertoli. II. Héterochromosome et mitoses de l'épithelium séminal). *Arch Biol* 27:93, 147–149, 1912
13. Painter TS: The Y-chromosome in mammals. *Science* 53:503–504, 1921
14. Painter TS: The spermatogenesis of man. *Anat Rec* 23:129, 1922
15. Painter TS: Studies in mammalian spermatogenesis: II. The spermatogenesis of man. *J Exp Zool* 37:291–336, 1923
16. Sachs L: Sex-linkage and the sex chromosomes in man. *Ann Eugenics* 18:255–261, 1954
17. Tjio JH, Levan A: The chromosome number of man. *Hereditas* 42:1–6, 1956
18. Hsu T-C: *Human and Mammalian Cytogenetics: An Historical Perspective.* New York, Springer-Verlag, 1979
19. Belling J: On counting chromosomes in pollen mother cells. *Am Naturalist* 55:573–574, 1921
20. Blakeslee AF, Avery AG: Methods of inducing doubling of chromosomes in plants. *J Hered* 28:392–411, 1937
21. Levan A: The effect of colchicine on root mitoses in allium. *Hereditas* 24:371–486, 1938
22. Slifer EH: Insect development: VI. The behavior of grasshopper embryos in anisotonic, balanced salt solutions. *J Exp Zool* 67:137–157, 1934

23. Hughes A: Some effects of abnormal tonicity on dividing cells in chick tissue cultures. Q J Microscop Sci 93:207–219, 1952
24. Makino S, Nishimura I: Water-pretreatment squash technic: A new and simple practical method for the chromosome study of animals. *Stain Technol* 27:1–7, 1952
25. Hsu T-C: Mammalian chromosomes in vitro: I. The karyotype of man. *J Hered* 43:172, 1952
26. Hsu T-C: Chromosomal evolution in cell populations. *Int Rev Cytol* 12:69–161, 1961
27. Court-Brown WM: Preface. In *Human Population Cytogenetics*. Amsterdam, North-Holland, 1967
28. Boveri T: Über mehrpolige Mitosen als Mittel zur Analyse des Zellkerns. *Verh Physikal-Med Ges* 35:67–88, 1902
29. Boveri T: *Zur Frage der Entwicklung maligner Tumoren*. Jena, Gustav Fischer-Verlag, 1914
30. Hsu T-C: A historical outline of the development of cancer cytogenetics. *Cancer Genet Cytogenet* 28:5–26, 1987
31. Waardenburg PJ: *Das menschliche Auge und seine Erbanlagen: Bibliographia Genetica VII*. The Hague, Netherlands, Martinus Nijhoff, 1932
32. Lejeune J, Gautier M, Turpin R: Étude des chromosomes somatiques de neuf enfants mongoliens. *Acad Sci (Paris) C R* 248:1721–1722, 1959
33. Caspersson T, Zech L, Modest EJ, et al: Chemical differentiation with fluorescent alkylating agents in *Vicia faba* metaphase chromosomes. *Exp Cell Res* 58:128–140, 1969
34. Caspersson T, Zech L, Johanson C: Differential banding of alkylating fluorochromes in human chromosomes. *Exp Cell Res* 60:315–319, 1970
35. Sumner AT, Evans HJ, Buckland RA: A new technique for distinguishing between human chromosomes. *Nature New Biol* 232:31–32, 1971
36. Patil SR, Merrick S, Lubs HA: Identification of each human chromosome with a modified Giemsa stain. *Science* 173:821–822, 1971
37. Drets ME, Shaw MW: Specific banding patterns of human chromosomes. *Proc Natl Acad Sci USA* 68:2073–2077, 1971
38. Arrighi FE, Hsu T-C: Localization of heterochromatin in human chromosomes. *Cytogenetics* 10:81–86, 1971
39. Chen TR, Ruddle FH: Karyotype analysis utilizing differentially stained constitutive heterochromatin of human and murine chromosomes. *Chromosoma* 34:51–72, 1971
40. Yunis G, Yasmineh WG: Heterochromatin, satellite DNA and cell function. *Science* 174:1200–1209, 1971
41. Benn PA, Perle MA: Chromosome staining and banding techniques. In *Human Cytogenetics: A Practical Approach*, Rooney DE, Czepulkowski BH (eds.). Oxford, IRL Press, pp. 57–84, 1986
42. Dutrillaux B, Lejeune J: Sur une nouvelle technique d'analyse du caryotype humain. *C R Acad Sci [III]* 272:2638–2640, 1971
43. Seabright M: A rapid banding technique for human chromosomes. *Lancet* 2:971–972, 1971

44. Wang HC, Fedoroff S: Banding in human chromosomes treated with trypsin. *Nature New Biol* 235:52–54, 1972
45. Yunis JJ: High resolution of human chromosomes. *Science* 191:1268–1270, 1976
46. Sandberg AA: Application of cytogenetics in neoplastic diseases. *CRC Crit Rev Clin Lab Sci* 22:219–274, 1985
47. Rowley JD: Finding order in chaos. *Perspect Biol Med* 32:371–384, 1989
48. Sandberg AA: Cytogenetic data and prognosis in acute leukemia. In *Therapy of Acute Leukemias*, Mandelli F, Amadori S, Mariani G (eds.). Proceedings of an international meeting, Rome, December 6–8, 1973, Lombardo Editore, pp. 186–192, 1977
49. Tjio JH, Nichols WW: History and present status of human chromosome studies. *In Vitro Cell Dev Biol* 21:305–313, 1985
50. Manolov G, Manolova Y: Marker band in one chromosome 14 from Burkitt lymphomas. *Nature* 237:33–34, 1972
51. Zech L, Hagland U, Nilsson K, et al: Characteristic chromosome abnormalities in biopsies and lymphoid-cell lines from patients with Burkitt and non-Burkitt lymphomas. *Int J Cancer* 17:47–56, 1976
52. Dofuku R, Biedler JL, Spengler BH, et al: Trisomy of chromosome 15 in spontaneous leukemia of AKR mice. *Proc Natl Acad Sci USA* 72:1515–1517, 1975
53. Third International Workshop on Chromosomes in Leukemia (Felix Mitelman, workshop organizer). *Cancer Genet Cytogenet* 4:95–142, 1981
54. Mitelman F: Catalogue of chromosome aberrations in cancer. *Cytogenet Cell Genet* 36:5–515, 1983
55. Cruciger QVJ, Pathak S, Cailleau R: Human breast carcinomas: Marker chromosomes involving 1q in seven cases. *Cytogenet Cell Genet* 17:231–235, 1976
56. Trujillo J, Cork A, Hart JS, et al: Clinical implications of aneuploid cytogenetic profiles in adult acute leukemia. *Cancer* 33:824–834, 1974
57. Fourth International Workshop on Chromosomes in Leukemia (September 1982). *Cancer Genet Cytogenet* 11:249–360, 1984
58. Yunis JJ, Bloomfield CD, Ensrud K: All cases of acute non-lymphocytic leukemia may have a chromosomal defect. *N Engl J Med* 305:135–139, 1981
59. Rowley JD: Chromosome changes in acute leukemia. *Br J Haematol* 44:339–346, 1980
60. Rowley JD: Identification of a translocation with quinacrine fluorescence in a patient with acute leukemia. *Ann Genet* 16:109–112, 1973
61. Trujillo JM, Cork A, Ahearn MJ, et al: Hematologic and cytologic characterization of 8/21 translocation acute granulocytic leukemia. *Blood* 53:695–706, 1979
62. Freireich EJ: Hematologic malignancies: Adult acute leukemia. *Hosp Pract* 21:91–110, 1986
63. Arthur DC, Bloomfield CD: Partial deletion of the long arm of chromosome 16 and bone marrow eosinophilia in acute nonlymphocytic leukemia: A new association. *Blood* 61:994–998, 1983

64. LeBeau MM, Larson RA, Bitter MA, et al: Association of an inversion of chromosome 16 with abnormal marrow eosinophils in acute myelomonocytic leukemia: A unique cytogenetic-clinicopathological association. *N Engl J Med* 309:630–636, 1983
65. Pearson M, Rowley JD: The relation of oncogenesis and cytogenetics in leukemia and lymphoma. *Annu Rev Med* 36:471–483, 1985
66. Freireich EJ: New strategies in the treatment of acute leukemia. *Acta Haematol* 78(Suppl 1):116–119, 1987
67. Golomb HM, Rowley JD, Vardiman J, et al: Partial deletion of long arm of chromosome 17: A specific abnormality in acute promyelocytic leukemia? *Arch Intern Med* 136:825–828, 1976
68. Rowley JD, Golomb HM, Vardiman J, et al: Further evidence for a nonrandom chromosomal abnormality in acute promyelocytic leukemia. *Int J Cancer* 20:869–872, 1977
69. Larson RA, Kondo K, Vardiman JW, et al: Every patient with acute promyelocytic leukemia may have a 15;17 translocation. *Am J Med* 76:827–841, 1984
70. Harrison CJ: Diagnosis of malignancy from chromosome preparations. In *Human Cytogenetics: A Practical Approach*, Rooney DE, Czepulkowski BH (eds.). Oxford, IRL Press, pp. 135–161, 1986
71. Philip P, Wantzin GL, Jensen MK, et al: Trisomy 8 in acute myeloid leukemia: A non-random event. *Scand J Haematol* 18:163–169, 1977
72. Ruutu P, Ruutu T, Vuopio P, et al: Defective chemotaxis in monosomy–7. *Nature* 265:146–147, 1977
73. Borgström GH, Teerenhovi L, Vuopio P, et al: 7 Monosomy in acute non-lymphocytic leukaemia: A cytogenetical and clinical study. Presented at the Symposium on Chromosomes et Hémopathies Malignes, Réunions Satellites du Congrès de Paris de la Société Internationale d'Hématologie, Centre Hospitalo, Universitaire de Poitiers, July 30–August 1, 1978
74. Rowley JD, Golomb HM, Vardiman J: Nonrandom chromosomal abnormalities in acute nonlymphocytic leukemia in patients treated for Hodgkin disease and non-Hodgkin lymphomas. *Blood* 50:759–770, 1977
75. Rowley JD: Leukemia as a second malignancy. Presented at the Symposium on Chromosomes et Hémopathies Malignes, Réunions Satellites du Congrès de Paris de la Société Internationale d'Hématologie, Centre Hospitalo, Universitaire de Poitiers, July 30–August 1, 1978
76. Keating MJ, Cork A, Broach Y, et al: Toward a clinically relevant cytogenetic classification of acute myelogenous leukemia. *Leuk Res* 11:119–133, 1987
77. Secker-Walker LM: The prognostic implications of chromosomal findings in acute lymphoblastic leukemia. *Cancer Genet Cytogenet* 11:233–248, 1984
78. Oshimura M, Freeman AI, Sandberg AA: Chromosomes and causation of human cancer and leukemia: XXVI. Banding studies in acute lymphoblastic leukemia (ALL). *Cancer* 40:1161–1172, 1977
79. Cimino MC, Rowley JD, Kinnealey A, et al: Banding studies of chro-

mosomal abnormalities in patients with acute lymphocytic leukemia. *Cancer Res* 39:227–238, 1979

80. Heim S, Mitelman F: Primary chromosome abnormalities in human neoplasia. *Adv Cancer Res* 52:1–43, 1989

81. Nowell PC: Chromosomal and molecular clues to tumor progression. *Semin Oncol* 16:116–127, 1989

82. Leder P, Battey J, Lenoir G, et al: Translocations among antibody genes in human cancer. *Science* 222:765–771, 1983

83. Williams DL, Look AT, Melvin SL: New chromosomal translocations correlate with specific immunophenotypes of childhood acute lymphoblastic leukemia. *Cell* 36:101–109, 1984

84. Propp S, Lizzi FA: Philadelphia chromosome in acute lymphocytic leukemia. *Blood* 36:353–360, 1970

85. Schmidt R, Dar H, Santorineou M, et al: Ph¹ chromosome and loss and reappearance of the Y chromosome in acute lymphocytic leukemia. *Lancet* 1:1145, 1975

86. Mandel EM, Shabtai F, Gafter U, et al: Ph¹-positive acute lymphocytic leukemia with chromosome 7 abnormalities. *Blood* 49:281–287, 1977

87. Ayraud N, Dujardin P, Audoly P: Leucémie aiguë lymphoblastique avec chromosome Philadelphie: Rôle probable d'une translocation 14–22. *Nouv Presse Med* 4:3013, 1975

88. Kurzrock R, Shtalrid M, Romero P, et al: A novel c-*abl* protein product in Philadelphia-positive acute lymphoblastic leukaemia. *Nature* 325:631–635, 1987

89. Catovsky D, Pittman S, O'Brien M, et al: Multiparameter studies in lymphoid leukemias. *Am J Clin Pathol* 72:736–745, 1979

90. Chan LC, Karhi KK, Rayter SI, et al: A novel *abl* protein expressed in Philadelphia chromosome positive acute lymphoblastic leukaemia. *Nature* 325:635–637, 1987

91. Clark SS, McLaughlin J, Crist WM, et al: Unique forms of the *abl* tyrosine kinase distinguish Ph¹-positive CML from Ph¹-positive ALL. *Science* 235:85–88, 1987

92. Williams DL, Tsiatis A, Barodeur GM, et al: Prognostic importance of chromosome number in 136 untreated children with acute lymphoblastic leukemia. *Blood* 60:864–871, 1982

93. Stass SA, Mirro J Jr: Lineage heterogeneity in acute leukaemia: Acute mixed-lineage leukaemia and lineage switch. *Clin Haematol* 15:811–827, 1986

94. Priest JR, Robison LL, McKenna RW, et al: Philadelphia chromosome positive childhood acute lymphoblastic leukemia. *Blood* 56:15–22, 1980

95. Pinkel D: Curing children of leukemia. *Accomplishments Cancer Res* 2:57–72, 1986

96. Dewald GW, Noel P, Dahl RJ, et al: Chromosome abnormalities in malignant hematologic disorders. *Proc Mayo Clin* 60:675–689, 1985

97. Land H, Parada LF, Weinberg RA: Cellular oncogenes and multistep carcinogenesis. *Science* 222:771–778, 1983

98. Gallucci BB: Selected concepts of cancer as a disease: From 1900 to oncogenes. *Oncol Nursing Forum* 12:69–78, 1985
99. Bishop JM: Cancer genes come of age. *Cell* 32:1018–1020, 1983
100. Stehelin D, Varmus HE, Bishop JM, et al: DNA related to the transforming gene(s) of avian sarcoma viruses is present in normal avian DNA. *Nature* 260:170–173, 1976
101. Cooper GM: Cellular transforming genes. *Science* 217:801–806, 1982
102. Cold Spring Harbor Laboratory: Origins of contemporary RNA tumor virus research. In *Molecular Biology of Tumor Viruses*, vol. 1, Weiss R, Teich N, Varmus H, Coffin J (eds.). New York, Cold Spring Harbor, pp. 1–24, 1982
103. Rous P: A sarcoma of the fowl transmissible by an agent separable from the tumor cells. *J Exp Med* 13:397–411, 1911
104. Watson JD, Tooze J, Kurtz DT: *Recombinant DNA: A Short Course.* New York, W.H. Freeman, 1983
105. Weinberg RA: Fewer and fewer oncogenes. *Cell* 30:3–4, 1982

9. Recombinant DNA and Human Molecular Analysis

1. Chargaff E: Preface to a grammar of biology: A hundred years of nucleic acid research. *Science* 172:637–642, 1971
2. Miescher F: *Die histochemischen und physiologischen Arbeiten.* Leipzig, Vogel, 1897
3. Lear J: *Recombinant DNA: The Untold Story.* New York, Crown, 1978
4. Watson JD, Tooze J, Kurtz DT: *Recombinant DNA: A Short Course.* New York, W.H. Freeman, 1983
5. Griffith F: The significance of pneumococcal types. *J Hyg (Lond)* 27:113–159, 1928
6. Avery OT, MacLeod CM, McCarty M: Studies on the chemical nature of the substance inducing transformation of pneumococcal types: Induction of transformation by a desoxyribonucleic acid fraction isolated from *Pneumococcus* type III. *J Exp Med* 79:137–157, 1944
7. Pollock MR: The discovery of DNA: An ironic tale of chance, prejudice and insight. *J Gen Microbiol* 63:1–20, 1970
8. Editor's comments: Nobel Prize for medicine. *Br Med J* 2:1114, 1962
9. Shorter E: *The Health Century.* New York, Doubleday, pp. 78–100, 1987
10. Pauling L, Itano HA, Singer SJ, et al: Sickle cell anemia: A molecular disease. *Science* 110:543–548, 1949
11. Asimov I: Amino acid aids dinosaur theory. *Houston Chronicle*, p. B5, July 3, 1989
12. Sanger F: Fractionation of oxidized insulin. *Biochem J* 44:126–128, 1949
13. Sanger F, Tuppy H: The amino-acid sequence in the phenylalanyl chain of insulin: 1. The identification of lower peptides from partial hydrolysates. *Biochem J* 49:463–481, 1951
14. Sanger F, Tuppy H: The amino-acid sequence in the phenylalanyl chain of insulin: 2. The investigation of peptides from enzymic hydrolysates. *Biochem J* 49:481–490, 1951
15. Sanger F, Thompson EOP: The amino-acid sequence in the glycyl chain

of insulin: I. The identification of lower peptides from partial hydrolysates. *Biochem J* 53:353–374, 1953

16. Chargaff E: Chemical specificity of nucleic acids and mechanism of their enzymatic degradation. *Experientia* 6:201–209, 1950

17. Chargaff E: Structure and function of nucleic acids as cell constituents. *Fed Proc* 10:654–659, 1951

18. Brown DM, Todd AR: Nucleotides: Part X. Some observations on the structure and chemical behaviour of the nucleic acids. *J Chem Soc* 1:52–58, 1952

19. Todd A: Nucleic acids and their role in future chemotherapy of tumours and virus diseases. *Br Med J* 2:517–522, 1959

20. D'Herelle F: *Le bactériophage: Son rôle dans l'immunité.* Paris, Masson et Cie, 1921

21. D'Herelle F: *Le bactériophage et son comportement.* Paris, Masson et Cie, 1926

22. Delbrück M, Delbrück MB: Bacterial viruses and sex. *Sci Am* 179:47–51, 1948

23. Hershey AD, Chase M: Independent functions of viral protein and nucleic acid in growth of bacteriophage. *J Gen Physiol* 36:39–56, 1953

24. Pauling L, Corey RB: Structure of the nucleic acids. *Nature* 171:346, 1953

25. Watson JD, Crick FHC: Molecular structure of nucleic acids: A structure for deoxyribose nucleic acid. *Nature* 171:737–738, 1953

26. Wilkins MHF, Stokes AR, Wilson HR: Molecular structure of deoxypentose nucleic acids. *Nature* 171:738–740, 1953

27. Kornberg A, Lehman IR, Simms ES: Polydesoxyribonucleotide synthesis by enzymes from *Escherichia coli. Fed Proc* 15:291–292, 1956

28. Kornberg A, Lehman IR, Bessman MJ, et al: Enzymic synthesis of deoxyribonucleic acid. *Biochim Biophys Acta* 21:197–198, 1956

29. Kornberg A: The synthesis of DNA. *Sci Am* 219(4):64–78, 1968

30. Lwoff A: Lysogeny. *Bact Rev* 17:269–337, 1953

31. Lwoff A: *Control and Interrelations of Metabolic and Viral Diseases of Bacteria.* Harvey Lecture, series 50 (1954–55). New York, Academic Press, pp. 92–111, 1955

32. Meselson M, Stahl FW: The replication of DNA in *Escherichia coli. Proc Natl Acad Sci USA* 44:671–682, 1958

33. Editor's comments: At the core of cancer and viruses. *Br Med J* 1:1519–1520, 1959

34. Jacob F, Monod J: Genetic regulatory mechanisms in the synthesis of proteins. *J Mol Biol* 3:318–356, 1961

35. Schlessinger BS, Schlessinger JH: *The Who's Who of Nobel Prize Winners.* Phoenix, AZ, Oryx Press, 1986

36. National Library of Medicine Sesquicentennial Commemorative Award, 1836–1986: *Tribute to America's Nobel Laureates in Medicine, Physiology and Chemistry,* 1986

37. Nirenberg MW, Matthaei JH: The dependence of cell-free protein synthesis in *E. coli* upon naturally occurring or synthetic polyribonucleotides. *Proc Natl Acad Sci USA* 47:1588–1602, 1961

38. Nobel Prizes for Medicine, 1968. *Nature* 220:324–325, 1968

39. Khorana HG: Synthesis of nucleotides, nucleotide coenzymes and polynucleotides. *Fed Proc* 19:931–941, 1960
40. Holley RW: Large-scale preparation of yeast "soluble" ribonucleic acid. *Biochem Biophys Res Commun* 10:186–188, 1963
41. Holley RW, Everett GA, Madison JT, et al: Nucleotide sequences in the yeast alanine transfer ribonucleic acid. *J Biol Chem* 240:2122–2128, 1965
42. Holley RW: The nucleotide sequence of a nucleic acid. *Sci Am* 214:30–39, 1966
43. Gefter ML, Becker A, Hurwitz J: The enzymatic repair of DNA: I. Formation of circular lambda DNA. *Proc Natl Acad Sci USA* 58:240–247, 1967
44. Olivera BM, Lehman IR: Linkage of polynucleotides through phosphodiester bonds by an enzyme from *Escherichia coli*. *Proc Natl Acad Sci USA* 57:1426–1433, 1967
45. Weiss B, Richardson CC: Enzymatic breakage and joining of deoxyribonucleic acid: I. Repair of single-strand breaks in DNA by an enzyme system from *Escherichia coli* infected with T4 bacteriophage. *Proc Natl Acad Sci USA* 57:1021–1028, 1967
46. Zimmerman SB, Little JW, Oshinsky CK, et al: Enzymatic joining of DNA strands: A novel reaction of diphosphopyridine nucleotide. *Proc Natl Acad Sci USA* 57:1841–1848, 1967
47. Cozzarelli NR, Melechen NE, Jovin TM, et al: Polynucleotide cellulose as a substrate for a polynucleotide ligase induced by phage T4. *Biochem Biophys Res Commun* 28:578–586, 1967
48. Sgaramella V, van de Sande JH, Khorana HG: Studies on polynucleotides: C. A novel joining reaction catalyzed by the T4-polynucleotide ligase. *Proc Natl Acad Sci USA* 67:1468–1475, 1970
49. Smith HO, Wilcox KW: A restriction enzyme from *Hemophilus influenzae*. *J Mol Biol* 51:379–391, 1970
50. Yoshimori RN: Ph.D. thesis, University of California San Francisco Medical Center, 1971
51. Boyer HW, Roulland-Dussoix D: A complementation analysis of the restriction and modification of DNA in *Escherichia coli*. *J Mol Biol* 41:459–472, 1969
52. Boyer HW: DNA restriction and modification mechanisms in bacteria. *Annu Rev Microbiol* 25:153–176, 1971
53. Boyer HW, Chow LT, Dugaiczyk A, et al: DNA substrate site for the Eco_{RII} restriction endonuclease and modification methylase. *Nature New Biol* 244:40–43, 1973
54. Mertz JE, Davis RW: Cleavage of DNA by R_1 restriction endonuclease generates cohesive ends. *Proc Natl Acad Sci USA* 69:3370–3374, 1972
55. Lobban PE, Kaiser AD: Enzymatic end-to-end joining of DNA molecules. *J Mol Biol* 78:453–471, 1973
56. Jackson DA, Symons RH, Berg P: Biochemical method for inserting new genetic information into DNA of simian virus 40: Circular SV40 DNA molecules containing lambda phage genes and the galactose operon of *Escherichia coli*. *Proc Natl Acad Sci USA* 69:2904–2909, 1972

57. Kato K-I, Gonçalves JM, Houts GE, et al: Deoxynucleotide-polymerizing enzymes of calf thymus gland: II. Properties of the terminal deoxynucleotidyltransferase. *J Biol Chem* 242:2780–2789, 1967

58. Denniston KJ, Enquist LW: Editors' comments. In *Recombinant DNA*. Stroudsburg, PA, Dowden, Hutchinson, & Ross, pp. 7–12, 1981

59. Cohen SN, Chang ACY, Hsu L: Nonchromosomal antibiotic resistance in bacteria: Genetic transformation of *Escherichia coli* by R-factor DNA. *Proc Natl Acad Sci USA* 69:2110–2114, 1972

60. Cohen SN, Chang ACY, Boyer HW, et al: Construction of biologically functional bacterial plasmids in vitro. *Proc Natl Acad Sci USA* 70:3240–3244, 1973

61. Chargaff E: Letter to the editors. *Science* 192:938–940, 1976

62. Fiers W, Contreras R, Duerinck F, et al: Complete nucleotide sequence of bacteriophage MS2 RNA: Primary and secondary structure of the replicase gene. *Nature* 260:500–507, 1976

63. Fiers W, Contreras R, Haegeman G, et al: Complete nucleotide sequence of SV40 DNA. *Nature* 273:113–120, 1978

64. Editor's comments: Viral RNA-dependent DNA polymerase. *Nature* 226:1209, 1970

65. Baltimore D: RNA-dependent DNA polymerase in virions of RNA tumour viruses. *Nature* 226:1209–1211, 1970

66. Temin HM, Mizutani S: RNA-dependent DNA polymerase in virions of Rous sarcoma virus. *Nature* 226:1211–1213, 1970

67. Havron D: The Nobelists. *Medical Tribune*, pp. 48–49, May 7, 1980

68. Itakura K, Hirose T, Crea R, et al: Expression in *Escherichia coli* of a chemically synthesized gene for the hormone somatostatin. *Science* 198:1056–1063, 1977

69. Goeddel DV, Kleid DG, Bolivar F, et al: Expression in *Escherichia coli* of chemically synthesized genes for human insulin. *Proc Natl Acad Sci USA* 76:106–110, 1979

70. Goeddel DV, Heyneker HL, Hozumi T, et al: Direct expression in *Escherichia coli* of a DNA sequence coding for human growth hormone. *Nature* 281:544–548, 1979

71. Gutterman JU, Fine S, Quesada J, et al: Recombinant leukocyte A interferon: Pharmacokinetics, single-dose tolerance, and biologic effects in cancer patients. *Ann Intern Med* 96:549–556, 1982

72. Taniguchi T, Sakai M, Fujii-Kuriyama Y, et al: Construction and identification of a bacterial plasmid containing the human fibroblast interferon gene sequence. *Proc Jpn Acad* 55(B):464–469, 1979

73. Yelverton E, Goeddel DV: Bacterial production of human leukocyte interferon. *Tex Rep Biol Med* 41:192–197, 1981–82

74. Taniguchi T, Guarente L, Roberts TM, et al: Expression of the human fibroblast interferon gene in *Escherichia coli*. *Proc Natl Acad Sci USA* 77:5230–5233, 1980

75. Derynck R, Content J, DeClercq E, et al: Isolation and structure of a human fibroblast interferon gene. *Nature* 285:542–547, 1980

76. Derynck R, Remaut E, Saman E, et al: Expression of human fibroblast interferon gene in *Escherichia coli. Nature* 287:193–197, 1980
77. Goeddel DV, Shepard HM, Yelverton E, et al: Synthesis of human fibroblast interferon by *E. coli. Nucleic Acids Res* 8:4057–4074, 1980
78. Nagata S, Taira H, Hall A, et al: Synthesis in *E. coli* of a polypeptide with human leukocyte interferon activity. *Nature* 284:316–320, 1980
79. Secher DS, Burke DC: A monoclonal antibody for large-scale purification of human leukocyte interferon. *Nature* 285:446–450, 1980
80. Gray PW, Leung DW, Pennica D, et al: Expression of human immune interferon cDNA in *E. coli* and monkey cells. *Nature* 295:503–508, 1982
81. Devos R, Cheroutre H, Taya Y, et al: Molecular cloning of human immune interferon cDNA and its expression in eukaryotic cells. *Nucleic Acids Res* 10:2487–2501, 1982
82. Pestka S: The purification and manufacture of human interferons. *Sci Am* 249:37–43, 1983
83. Kan YW, Dozy AM: Antenatal diagnosis of sickle-cell anaemia by D.N.A. analysis of amniotic-fluid cells. *Lancet* 2:910–911, 1978
84. Beebe TP Jr, Wilson TE, Ogletree DF, et al: Direct observation of native DNA structures with the scanning tunneling microscope. *Science* 243:370–372, 1989
85. Asimov I: First look at DNA proves revealing. *Houston Chronicle,* p. B6, February 20, 1989
86. Culliton BJ: Gene test begins. *Science* 244:913, 1989
87. Culliton BJ: Fighting cancer with designer cells. *Science* 244:1430–1433, 1989
88. Arias R, Breu G: A medical breakthrough gives new hope to David Reitz—and all kids with cystic fibrosis. *People Magazine,* pp. 83–89, September 11, 1989

10. Future Directions

1. Pinkel D: Curing children of leukemia. *Accomplishments Cancer Res* 2:57–72, 1986
2. Farber S, Diamond LK, Mercer RD, et al: Temporary remissions in acute leukemia in children prolonged by folic acid antagonist, 4-aminopteroylglutamic acid (aminopterin). *N Engl J Med* 238:787–793, 1948
3. Knudson AG Jr: Mutation and cancer: Statistical study of retinoblastoma. *Proc Natl Acad Sci USA* 68:820–823, 1971
4. Hsu T-C: Genetic predisposition to cancer with special reference to mutagen sensitivity. *In Vitro Cell Dev Biol* 23:591–603, 1987
5. Yarbro JW: The new biology of cancer: Future clinical applications. *Semin Oncol* 16:254–259, 1989
6. Land H, Parada LF, Weinberg RA: Cellular oncogenes and multistep carcinogenesis. *Science* 222:771–778, 1983
7. Nowell PC: Chromosomal and molecular clues to tumor progression. *Semin Oncol* 16:116–127, 1989
8. Brandt SJ, Peters WP, Atwater SK, et al: Effect of recombinant human

granulocyte-macrophage colony-stimulating factor on hematopoietic reconstitution after high dose of chemotherapy and autologous bone marrow transplantation. *N Engl J Med* 318:869–876, 1988

9. Morstyn G, Burgess AW: Hemopoietic growth factors: A review. *Cancer Res* 48:5624–5637, 1988

10. Barlow DP, Bucan M, Lehrach H, et al: Close genetic and physical linkage between the murine haemopoietic growth factor genes GM-CSF and multi-CSF (IL–3). *Eur Mol Biol Organization J* 6:617–623, 1987

11. Huebner K, Isobe M, Croce CM, et al: The human gene encoding GM-CSF is at 5q21-q32, the chromosome region deleted in the 5q-anomaly. *Science* 230:1282–1285, 1985

12. Pettenati MJ, LeBeau MM, Lemons RS, et al: Assignment of CSF–1 to 5q33.1: Evidence for clustering of genes regulating hematopoiesis and for their involvement in the deletion of the long arm of chromosome 5 in myeloid disorders. *Proc Natl Acad Sci USA* 84:2970–2974, 1987

Permissions/Credits

Sources of Quotations

T. S. Eliot, excerpt from "Little Gidding" in *Four Quartets*, copyright 1943 by T. S. Eliot and renewed 1971 by Esme Valerie Eliot. Reprinted by permission of Harcourt Brace Jovanovich, Inc., and Faber and Faber Ltd., London.

Hilaire Belloc, "Physicians of the Utmost Fame." Reprinted by permission of Alfred A. Knopf, Inc.

Robert Frost, "The Secret Sits." From *The Poetry of Robert Frost*, edited by Edward Connery Lathem. Copyright 1942 by Robert Frost, copyright 1969 by Holt, Rinehart and Winston, copyright 1970 by Lesley Frost Ballantine. Reprinted by permission of Henry Holt and Company, Inc., and Jonathan Cape Ltd., London.

Emily Dickinson, " 'Hope' is the thing with feathers." From *The Complete Poems of Emily Dickinson*, edited by Thomas H. Johnson. Reprinted by permission of Little, Brown and Company.

Candace Galen, "Diversity's the Splice of Life." From *Perspectives in Biology and Medicine* 25(3):453, 1982. Reprinted by permission of the editor of that journal and Dr. Galen.

William Faulkner quotation from Ruel E. Foster, "Faulkner's Late Migration to a Pleasant Life among the 'Snobs.' " *The National Observer*, p. 22, February 3, 1964.

Photograph Credits

Page

2   From Thorburn AL: Alfred Francois Donné, 1801–1878, discoverer of *Trichomonas vaginalis* and of leukemia. *Br J Venereal Dis* 50:377–380, 1974. Courtesy of the editor of the journal, the British Medical Association, and Dr. Thorburn's widow

4   (*Left*) From Damon HF: Leucocythemia: An essay (Awarded the Boylston Medical Prize of Harvard University for 1863; Boston, DeVries, Ibarra and Company, 1864). In Rosenthal N: The lymphomas and leukemias. *Bull NY Acad Med* 30:583–600, 1954. Courtesy of the New York Academy of Medicine

4   (*Right*) From Rosenthal N: The lymphomas and leukemias. *Bull NY Acad Med* 30:583–600, 1954. Courtesy of the New York Academy of Medicine

5   From *Der Internist* 10:79, 1969. Courtesy of Springer-Verlag, Heidelberg

19   Courtesy of Dr. Peter C. Nowell

31   From Holland JF: Breaking the cure barrier. *J Clin Oncol* 1:75–90, 1983. Courtesy of Dr. Holland and W.B. Saunders Company

34   From Parascandola J: Carl Voegtlin and the "arsenic receptor" in chemotherapy. *J Hist Med Allied Sci* 32:151–171, 1977. Courtesy of the editor of that journal and of the National Library of Medicine

40 & 41   Courtesy of Professor Norbert Brock

46   From Pochedly C: Dr. James A. Wolff: II. First successful chemotherapy of acute leukemia. *Am J Pediatr Hematol Oncol* 6:449–454, 1984. Courtesy of Dr. Pochedly and Raven Press

108   Courtesy of John Hammarley and the Oregon Health Sciences University

143   Courtesy of Elizabeth Hutchins, daughter of Theophilus S. Painter

146   Courtesy of Joe Hin Tjio

Subject Index

ABVD regimen, 81
Acute leukemia: Adriamycin therapy, 60–61; AMSA therapy, 61–63; Ara-C therapy, 49–53; cyclophosphamide therapy, 40; cytogenetic abnormalities, 151–58; effects of chemotherapy (1961), 77; etoposide therapy, 64–65; first description of, 6; interferon therapy, 127–30; NCI cooperative trials, 76–77; teniposide therapy, 64–65; vincristine therapy, 57–58. *See also specific diagnoses*
Acute Leukemia Task Force, 77–78
Acute lymphocytic leukemia (ALL): Adriamycin therapy, 60–61; AMSA therapy, 62–63; Ara-C therapy, 50, 53; L-asparaginase therapy, 54–55; BCG therapy, 122–23; B cell ALL, 132, 157–58; *bcr-abl* hybrid gene, 158; curative chemotherapy, 70; daunomycin therapy, 59; effects of chemotherapy (1961), 77; etoposide therapy, 64–65; first efforts for cure of, 77–78; ifosfamide therapy, 42–44; incidence of secondary AML, 65; interferon therapy, 128; interleukin 2 pretreatment, 132; karyotypic patterns, 156–58; meningeal leukemia, 83–85; 6-mercaptopurine therapy, 48, 73; methotrexate therapy, 47, 123; mitoxantrone therapy,

67; NCI cooperative trials, 76–77; Philadelphia chromosome in, 21, 157–58; teniposide therapy, 64–65; "total therapy," 80; vincaleukoblastine therapy, 57; vincristine therapy, 57–58
Acute monocytic leukemia, 9, 57, 64
Acute myelogenous leukemia (AML): Adriamycin therapy, 60–61; AMSA therapy, 61–63; Ara-C therapy, 50–53; L-asparaginase therapy, 55; BCG therapy, 123–24; bone marrow transplantation, 107–18; combination therapy using Ara-C, 51, 81–83; daunomycin therapy, 59; effects of chemotherapy (1961), 77; etoposide therapy, 64–65; ifosfamide therapy, 42–43; interferon therapy, 128; methyl-GAG therapy, 69; mitoxantrone therapy, 67; podophyllotoxin and secondary AML, 65; prognostic value of GM-CSF, 137; secondary to etoposide therapy, 65; secondary to therapy for Hodgkin's disease, 68; thioguanine therapy, 48; vincristine therapy, 57
Acute myelomonocytic leukemia, 64
Acute non-lymphocytic leukemia (ANLL): Ara-C therapy, 50–53; bone marrow transplantation, 107–18; karyotypic patterns, 154–56

Name Index